Teen Health Series

Mental Health Information
For Teens, Fifth Edition

Mental Health Information
For Teens, Fifth Edition

Health Tips About Mental Wellness
And Mental Illness

Including Facts About Recognizing And
Treating Mood, Anxiety, Personality, Psychotic,
Behavioral, Impulse Control, And Addiction Disorders

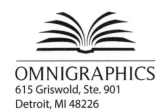

OMNIGRAPHICS
615 Griswold, Ste. 901
Detroit, MI 48226

Bibliographic Note
Because this page cannot legibly accommodate all the copyright notices, the Bibliographic Note portion of the Preface constitutes an extension of the copyright notice.

* * *

Omnigraphics
a part of Relevant Information
Siva Ganesh Maharaja, *Managing Editor*

* * *

Library of Congress Cataloging-in-Publication Data

Names: Omnigraphics, Inc., issuing body.

Title: Mental health information for teens: health tips about mental wellness and mental illness including facts about recognizing and treating mood, anxiety, personality, psychotic, behavioral, impulse control, and addiction disorders.

Description: Fifth edition. | Detroit, MI: Omnigraphics, [2017] | Series: Teen health series | Audience: Grade 9 to 12. | Includes bibliographical references and index.

Identifiers: LCCN 2017028218 (print) | LCCN 2017028950 (ebook) | ISBN 9780780815742 (eBook) | ISBN 9780780815735 (hardcover: alk. paper)

Subjects: LCSH: Teenagers--Mental health. | Adolescent psychology. | Child mental health.

Classification: LCC RJ499 (ebook) | LCC RJ499.M419 2017 (print) | DDC 616.8900835--dc23

LC record available at https://lccn.loc.gov/2017028218

This book is printed on acid-free paper meeting the ANSI Z39.48 Standard. The infinity symbol that appears above indicates that the paper in this book meets that standard.

Printed in the United States

Table Of Contents

Preface

Part One: Mental Health And Mental Illness

Part Two: Mood And Anxiety Disorders

Part Three: Personality And Psychotic Disorders

Part Four: Behavioral, Impulse Control, And Addiction Disorders

Part Five: Other Situations And Disorders With Mental Health Consequences

Part Six: Mental Health Treatments

Part Seven: Mental Wellness Topics For Teens

Part Eight: If You Need More Information

Preface

About This Book

Adolescence is difficult. Not only are teens under stress to be liked, do well in school, and get along with family, they must cope with hormonal changes and make important decisions about their lives. Stressors such as these are normal, but teens sometimes find themselves feeling sad, hopeless, overwhelmed, or worthless. At a certain point, these feelings are possible signs of debilitating mental health problems, and teens experiencing them are not alone. According to the Centers for Disease Control and Prevention (CDC), an estimated one in five adolescents suffer from some kind of mental disorder. However, less than half of them received any treatment for their medical condition.

Mental Health Information For Teens, Fifth Edition offers updated information on mental health and its importance. It presents facts about the causes, warning signs, and diagnosis of mental illnesses, and explains how the adolescent brain differs from the adult brain. Some of the specific disorders described in detail include anxiety, depression, eating disorders, posttraumatic stress disorder, psychoses, schizophrenia, and impulse control disorders. Mental health therapies—both traditional and alternative—are discussed, and the consequences of not receiving treatment are addressed. A section on mental wellness provides tips for building healthy self-esteem, coping with stress and disaster, getting along with family and friends, and dealing with challenges such as divorce, abuse, grief, and thoughts of suicide. For readers seeking more information, the book concludes with suggestions for additional reading, a list of crisis lines, and a directory of mental health organizations.

How To Use This Book

This book is divided into parts and chapters. Parts focus on broad areas of interest; chapters are devoted to single topics within a part.

Part One: Mental Health And Mental Illness offers information on understanding mental health, its overall effect on well-being, and how resilience plays a vital role in mental wellness. Mental illness is defined, and its possible causes and warning signs are described. A chapter on few mental health risks and protective factors are discussed.

Part Two: Mood And Anxiety Disorders discusses an array of disorders that alter emotional and fear responses. These include depression, premenstrual syndrome, seasonal affective disorder, bipolar disorder, generalized anxiety disorder, social anxiety disorder, obsessive-compulsive disorder, posttraumatic stress disorder, panic disorder, and phobias.

Part Three: Personality And Psychotic Disorders describes mental illnesses that affect how people perceive reality. These include antisocial disorders, borderline personality disorder, factitious disorders, and dissociative disorders, as well as psychosis and schizophrenia.

Part Four: Behavioral, Impulse Control, And Addiction Disorders explores mental illnesses that influence how people act and possibly disregard societal norms. Examples include eating disorders, body dysmorphic disorder, impulse control disorder, disruptive behavior disorders, and comorbidity.

Part Five: Other Situations And Disorders With Mental Health Consequences provides information on adolescent circumstances that may impact mental wellbeing. These include puberty, child maltreatment, bullying, violence, and self-harm. Chronic disorders that may impact mental health, including autism spectrum disorder, attention deficit hyperactivity disorder (ADHD), and Tourette syndrome, are also discussed.

Part Six: Mental Health Treatments explains how mental illness is diagnosed and the ways in which the treatment of children with mental illness can differ from that of adults. Various common approaches to mental healthcare—including psychotherapy, the use of medications, and complementary and alternative medicine practices—are also described.

Part Seven: Mental Wellness Topics For Teens offers information on coping with challenges that can arise during adolescence. It provides tips for building a healthy self-esteem, improving mental health, dealing with depression, and coping with stress. It also offers strategies for handling traumatic events, important relationships, and thoughts of suicide.

Part Eight: If You Need More Information offers suggestions for additional reading, a list of crisis helplines and hotlines, and a directory of organizations able to provide further materials about adolescent mental health.

Bibliographic Note

This volume contains documents and excerpts from publications issued by the following government agencies: Agency for Healthcare Research and Quality (AHRQ); Centers for Disease Control and Prevention (CDC); Child Welfare Information Gateway; ClinicalTrials.gov; Federal Occupational Health (FOH); National Cancer Institute (NCI); National Center for Complementary and Integrative Health (NCCIH); National Institute of Mental Health (NIMH); National Institute on Drug Abuse (NIDA); National Institute on Drug Abuse (NIDA) for Teens; *NIH News in Health*; Office of Disease Prevention and Health Promotion (ODPHP); Office of the Assistant Secretary for Preparedness and Response (ASPR); Office on Women's Health (OWH); Substance Abuse and Mental Health Services Administration (SAMHSA); U.S. Department of Health and Human Services (HHS); U.S. Department of Veterans Affairs (VA); and Youth.gov.

It may also contain original material produced by Omnigraphics and reviewed by medical consultants.

The photograph on the front cover is © Meg Wallace Photography/Shutterstock.

Medical Review

Omnigraphics contracts with a team of qualified, senior medical professionals who serve as medical consultants for the *Teen Health Series*. As necessary, medical consultants review reprinted and originally written material for currency and accuracy. Citations including the phrase, Reviewed (month, year)" indicate material reviewed by this team. Medical consultation services are provided to the *Teen Health Series* editors by:

Dr. Vijayalakshmi, MBBS, DGO, MD
Dr. Senthil Selvan, MBBS, DCH, MD
Dr. K. Sivanandham, MBBS, DCH, MS (Research), PhD

About The *Teen Health Series*

At the request of librarians serving today's young adults, the *Teen Health Series* was developed as a specially focused set of volumes within Omnigraphics' *Health Reference Series*. Each volume deals comprehensively with a topic selected according to the needs and interests of people in middle school and high school. Teens seeking preventive guidance, information about disease warning signs, medical statistics, and risk factors for health problems will find answers to their questions in the *Teen Health Series*. The *Series*, however, is not intended to serve as a tool for diagnosing illness, in prescribing treatments, or as a substitute for the physician/patient relationship. All people concerned about medical symptoms or the possibility of disease are encouraged to seek professional care from an appropriate healthcare provider.

If there is a topic you would like to see addressed in a future volume of the *Teen Health Series*, please write to:

Editor
Teen Health Series
Omnigraphics
615 Griswold, Ste. 901
Detroit, MI 48226

A Note About Spelling And Style

Teen Health Series editors use *Stedman's Medical Dictionary* as an authority for questions related to the spelling of medical terms and the *Chicago Manual of Style* for questions related to grammatical structures, punctuation, and other editorial concerns. Consistent adherence is not always possible, however, because the individual volumes within the *Series* include many documents from a wide variety of different producers and copyright holders, and the editor's primary goal is to present material from each source as accurately as is possible following the terms specified by each document's producer. This sometimes means that information in different chapters or sections may follow other guidelines and alternate spelling authorities.

Part One
Mental Health And Mental Illness

Chapter 1

Understanding Mental Health

Most of us feel sad, lonely, or anxious at times. That's just human. But sometimes people feel so sad, hopeless, worried, or worthless that they don't want to do things like get out of bed or go to school. These feelings can be signs that you need help for a mental health problem. Depression, anxiety, eating disorders, and other mental health issues can be treated. If you think you have a problem, talk to an adult you trust.

Talk to your parents or a trusted adult if you:

- Can't eat or sleep

- Can't do regular tasks like going to school

- Don't want to do things you used to enjoy

- Don't want to hang out with your friends or family

- Feel like you can't control your feelings and it's hurting your relationships

- Have low energy or no energy

- Feel hopeless

- Feel numb or like nothing matters

About This Chapter: Text in this chapter begins with excerpts from "Could I Have A Mental Health Problem?" girlshealth.gov, Office on Women's Health (OWH), January 7, 2015; Text beginning with the heading "What Is Mental Health?" is excerpted from "What Is Mental Health?" MentalHealth.gov, U.S. Department of Health and Human Services (HHS), May 31, 2013. Reviewed July 2017; Text under the heading "Impact Of Mental Health Disorders" is excerpted from "Module 3—Understanding Mental Disorders, Treatment, And Recovery," Substance Abuse and Mental Health Services Administration (SAMHSA), February 9, 2010. Reviewed July 2017; Text under the heading "Mental Health Myths And Facts" is excerpted from "Mental Health Myths And Facts," MentalHealth.gov, U.S. Department of Health and Human Services (HHS), May 31, 2013. Reviewed July 2017.

- Can't stop thinking about certain things or memories

- Often feel confused or forgetful

- Feel edgy, angry, upset, worried, or scared a lot

- Want to harm yourself or others

- Can't stop yourself from dieting or exercising a lot

- Have aches and pains that don't have a clear cause

- Hear voices

- Feel very sad for months after a loss or death

- Feel like your mind is being controlled or is out of control

What Is Mental Health?

Mental health includes our emotional, psychological, and social well-being. It affects how we think, feel, and act. It also helps determine how we handle stress, relate to others, and make choices. Mental health is important at every stage of life, from childhood and adolescence through adulthood.

Over the course of your life, if you experience mental health problems, your thinking, mood, and behavior could be affected. Many factors contribute to mental health problems, including:

- Biological factors, such as genes or brain chemistry

- Life experiences, such as trauma or abuse

- Family history of mental health problems

Mental health problems are common but help is available. People with mental health problems can get better and many recover completely.

Mental Health And Wellness

Positive mental health allows people to:

- Realize their full potential

- Cope with the stresses of life

- Work productively

- Make meaningful contributions to their communities

Ways to maintain positive mental health include:

- Getting professional help if you need it

- Connecting with others

- Staying positive

- Getting physically active

- Helping others

- Getting enough sleep

- Developing coping skills

Early Warning Signs Of Mental Illnesses

Not sure if you or someone you know is living with mental health problems? Experiencing one or more of the following feelings or behaviors can be an early warning sign of a problem:

- Eating or sleeping too much or too little

- Pulling away from people and usual activities

- Having low or no energy

- Feeling numb or like nothing matters

- Having unexplained aches and pains

- Feeling helpless or hopeless

- Smoking, drinking, or using drugs more than usual

- Feeling unusually confused, forgetful, on edge, angry, upset, worried, or scared

- Yelling or fighting with family and friends

- Experiencing severe mood swings that cause problems in relationships

- Having persistent thoughts and memories you can't get out of your head

- Hearing voices or believing things that are not true

- Thinking of harming yourself or others

- Inability to perform daily tasks like taking care of your kids or getting to work or school

You Are Not Alone

1/2 of teens have a mental health disorder at some point, according to a national survey. You can feel better! Mental health problems can be treated. Get help if you need it.

Impact Of Mental Health Disorders

- Thought processes, moods and emotions are affected by mental disorders.

- Mental disorders are biologically based.

- What matters most is the life impact.

- Disorders can be more, or less, serious, and may change over time.

- Cause is less important than current impact.

- Violence is not associated with all disorders.

Parent-reported information from the 2011-12 National Survey of Children's Health showed that 1 out of 7 U.S. children aged 2 to 8 years had a diagnosed mental, behavioral, or developmental disorder (MBDD). Many family, community, and healthcare factors were related to the children having MBDDs.

- Children with the following characteristics were more likely to have a MBDD:
  - Boys
  - Children age 6 to 8 years
  - Non-Hispanic white children
- Children were more likely to have a MBDD if they were from:
  - Poor families (those living at less than 100% of the federal poverty level) and
  - Families that spoke English in the home

(Source: "Children's Mental Health," Centers for Disease Control and Prevention (CDC).)

Mental Health Myths And Facts

Can you tell the difference between a mental health myth and fact? Learn the truth about the most common mental health myths.

Mental Health Problems Affect Everyone

Myth: Mental health problems don't affect me.

Fact: Mental health problems are actually very common. In 2014, about:

- One in five American adults experienced a mental health issue

- One in 10 young people experienced a period of major depression

- One in 25 Americans lived with a serious mental illness, such as schizophrenia, bipolar disorder, or major depression

Suicide is the 10th leading cause of death in the United States. It accounts for the loss of more than 41,000 American lives each year, more than double the number of lives lost to homicide.

Myth: Children don't experience mental health problems.

Fact: Even very young children may show early warning signs of mental health concerns. These mental health problems are often clinically diagnosable, and can be a product of the interaction of biological, psychological, and social factors.

Half of all mental health disorders show first signs before a person turns 14 years old, and three quarters of mental health disorders begin before age 24.

Unfortunately, less than 20 percent of children and adolescents with diagnosable mental health problems receive the treatment they need. Early mental health support can help a child before problems interfere with other developmental needs.

Myth: People with mental health problems are violent and unpredictable.

Fact: The vast majority of people with mental health problems are no more likely to be violent than anyone else. Most people with mental illness are not violent and only 3–5 percent of violent acts can be attributed to individuals living with a serious mental illness. In fact, people with severe mental illnesses are over 10 times more likely to be victims of violent crime than the general population. You probably know someone with a mental health problem and don't even realize it, because many people with mental health problems are highly active and productive members of our communities.

Myth: People with mental health needs, even those who are managing their mental illness, cannot tolerate the stress of holding down a job.

Fact: People with mental health problems are just as productive as other employees. Employers who hire people with mental health problems report good attendance and punctuality as well as motivation, good work, and job tenure on par with or greater than other employees.

When employees with mental health problems receive effective treatment, it can result in:

- Lower total medical costs
- Increased productivity
- Lower absenteeism
- Decreased disability costs

Myth: Personality weakness or character flaws cause mental health problems. People with mental health problems can snap out of it if they try hard enough.

Fact: Mental health problems have nothing to do with being lazy or weak and many people need help to get better. Many factors contribute to mental health problems, including:

- Biological factors, such as genes, physical illness, injury, or brain chemistry
- Life experiences, such as trauma or a history of abuse
- Family history of mental health problems

People with mental health problems can get better and many recover completely.

Helping Individuals With Mental Health Problems

Myth: There is no hope for people with mental health problems. Once a friend or family member develops mental health problems, he or she will never recover.

Fact: Studies show that people with mental health problems get better and many recover completely. Recovery refers to the process in which people are able to live, work, learn, and participate fully in their communities. There are more treatments, services, and community support systems than ever before, and they work.

Myth: Therapy and self-help are a waste of time. Why bother when you can just take a pill?

Fact: Treatment for mental health problems varies depending on the individual and could include medication, therapy, or both. Many individuals work with a support system during the healing and recovery process.

Myth: I can't do anything for a person with a mental health problem.

Fact: Friends and loved ones can make a big difference. Only 44 percent of adults with diagnosable mental health problems and less than 20 percent of children and adolescents receive needed treatment. Friends and family can be important influences to help someone get the treatment and services they need by:

- Reaching out and letting them know you are available to help

- Helping them access mental health services

- Learning and sharing the facts about mental health, especially if you hear something that isn't true

- Treating them with respect, just as you would anyone else

- Refusing to define them by their diagnosis or using labels such as "crazy"

Myth: Prevention doesn't work. It is impossible to prevent mental illnesses.

Fact: Prevention of mental, emotional, and behavioral disorders focuses on addressing known risk factors such as exposure to trauma that can affect the chances that children, youth, and young adults will develop mental health problems. Promoting the social-emotional well-being of children and youth leads to:

- Higher overall productivity

- Better educational outcomes

- Lower crime rates

- Stronger economies

- Lower healthcare costs

- Improved quality of life

- Increased lifespan

- Improved family life

Online Info

Websites and other online resources sometimes offer great support and tools for mental health. Sometimes, though, they actually promote poor habits. Your best bet is to work with an adult or ask your doctor about any online info.

Lots of help is available if you are having mental health problems. You can learn about therapy, and you can find a therapist near you. You can text for help with problems and contact a hotline if you're thinking about suicide. Your life can get so much better!

Teens who have faced mental health problems are connecting with each other through photos, videos, and more on OK2TALK (www.ok2talk.org). Read about their experiences and their stories of hope, strength, and recovery.

Chapter 2

The Teen Brain: Still Under Construction

One of the ways that scientists have searched for the causes of mental illness is by studying the development of the brain from birth to adulthood. Powerful new technologies have enabled them to track the growth of the brain and to investigate the connections between brain function, development, and behavior.

The research has turned up some surprises, among them the discovery of striking changes taking place during the teen years. These findings have altered long-held assumptions about the timing of brain maturation. In key ways, the brain doesn't look like that of an adult until the early 20s. An understanding of how the brain of an adolescent is changing may help explain a puzzling contradiction of adolescence: Young people at this age are close to a lifelong peak of physical health, strength, and mental capacity, and yet, for some, this can be a hazardous age. Mortality rates jump between early and late adolescence. Rates of death by injury between ages 15–19 are about six times that of the rate between ages 10–14. Crime rates are highest among young males and rates of alcohol abuse are high relative to other ages. Even though most adolescents come through this transitional age well, it's important to understand the risk factors for behavior that can have serious consequences. Genes, childhood experience, and the environment in which a young person reaches adolescence all shape behavior. Adding to this complex picture, research is revealing how all these factors act in the context of a brain that is changing, with its own impact on behavior.

The more we learn, the better we may be able to understand the abilities and vulnerabilities of teens, and the significance of this stage for life-long mental health.

About This Chapter: Text in this chapter begins with excerpts from "The Teen Brain: Still Under Construction," National Institute of Mental Health (NIMH), 2011. Reviewed July 2017; Text under heading "The Teen Brain: Six Things To Know" is excerpted from "The Teen Brain: 6 Things To Know," National Institute of Mental Health (NIMH), August 2016.

The "Visible" Brain

A clue to the degree of change taking place in the teen brain came from studies in which scientists did brain scans of children as they grew from early childhood through age 20. The scans revealed unexpectedly late changes in the volume of gray matter, which forms the thin, folding outer layer or cortex of the brain. The cortex is where the processes of thought and memory are based. Over the course of childhood, the volume of gray matter in the cortex increases and then declines. A decline in volume is normal at this age and is in fact a necessary part of maturation.

The assumption for many years had been that the volume of gray matter was highest in very early childhood, and gradually fell as a child grew. The more recent scans, however, revealed that the high point of the volume of gray matter occurs during early adolescence.

While the details behind the changes in volume on scans are not completely clear, the results push the timeline of brain maturation into adolescence and young adulthood. In terms of the volume of gray matter seen in brain images, the brain does not begin to resemble that of an adult until the early 20s.

The scans also suggest that different parts of the cortex mature at different rates. Areas involved in more basic functions mature first: those involved, for example, in the processing of information from the senses, and in controlling movement. The parts of the brain responsible for more "top-down" control, controlling impulses, and planning ahead—the hallmarks of adult behavior—are among the last to mature.

What's Gray Matter?

The details of what is behind the increase and decline in gray matter are still not completely clear. Gray matter is made up of the cell bodies of neurons, the nerve fibers that project from them, and support cells. One of the features of the brain's growth in early life is that there is an early blooming of synapses—the connections between brain cells or neurons—followed by pruning as the brain matures. Synapses are the relays over which neurons communicate with each other and are the basis of the working circuitry of the brain. Already more numerous than an adult's at birth, synapses multiply rapidly in the first months of life. A 2-year-old has about half again as many synapses as an adult. (For an idea of the complexity of the brain: A cube of brain matter, one millimeter on each side, can contain between 35 and 70 million neurons and an estimated 500 billion synapses.)

Scientists believe that the loss of synapses as a child matures is part of the process by which the brain becomes more efficient. Although genes play a role in the decline in synapses, animal research has shown that experience also shapes the decline. Synapses "exercised" by experience survive and are strengthened, while others are pruned away. Scientists are working to determine to what extent the changes in gray matter on brain scans during the teen years reflect growth and pruning of synapses.

A Spectrum Of Change

Research, using many different approaches, is showing that more than gray matter is changing in adolescence. Other changes include:

- Connections between different parts of the brain increase throughout childhood and well into adulthood. As the brain develops, the fibers connecting nerve cells are wrapped in a protein that greatly increases the speed with which they can transmit impulses from cell to cell. The resulting increase in connectivity—a little like providing a growing city with a fast, integrated communication system—shapes how well different parts of the brain work in tandem. Research is finding that the extent of connectivity is related to growth in intellectual capacities such as memory and reading ability.

- Several lines of evidence suggest that the brain circuitry involved in emotional responses is changing during the teen years. Functional brain imaging studies, for example, suggest that the responses of teens to emotionally loaded images and situations are heightened relative to younger children and adults. The brain changes underlying these patterns involve brain centers and signaling molecules that are part of the reward system with which the brain motivates behavior. These age-related changes shape how much different parts of the brain are activated in response to experience, and in terms of behavior, the urgency and intensity of emotional reactions.

- Enormous hormonal changes take place during adolescence. Reproductive hormones shape not only sex-related growth and behavior, but overall social behavior. Hormone systems involved in the brain's response to stress are also changing during the teens. As with reproductive hormones, stress hormones can have complex effects on the brain, and as a result, behavior.

- In terms of sheer intellectual power, the brain of an adolescent is a match for an adult's. The capacity of a person to learn will never be greater than during adolescence. At the same time, behavioral tests, sometimes combined with functional brain imaging, suggest differences in how adolescents and adults carry out mental tasks. Adolescents and adults seem to engage different parts of the brain to different extents during tests requiring calculation and impulse control, or in reaction to emotional content.

- Research suggests that adolescence brings with it brain-based changes in the regulation of sleep that may contribute to teens' tendency to stay up late at night. Along with the obvious effects of sleep deprivation, such as fatigue and difficulty maintaining attention, inadequate sleep is a powerful contributor to irritability and depression. Studies of children and adolescents have found that sleep deprivation can increase impulsive behavior; some researchers report finding that it is a factor in delinquency. Adequate sleep is central to physical and emotional health.

It's All About Hormones

During puberty, your brain releases various hormones that help your body to mature by producing testosterone (in boys) and estrogen (in girls). Resulting changes can go beyond physical development to include emotional and mood changes—although some researchers think mood swings may relate more to changes in the teen brain than to hormonal spurts.

Other important hormones also come into play in the teen years. Melatonin is a hormone that helps your body regulate sleep cycles by making you feel sleepy after the sun goes down. Melatonin levels in adolescents don't start to rise until about 10:30 p.m., which might explain why many teens want to stay up late despite their parents' wishes. Research shows that for adolescents, melatonin levels remain high, even after they wake up, which is why teens may feel sleepy in the morning.

Our bodies also release something called "stress hormones," such as cortisol. The stress hormone cortisol governs how well someone responds to or recovers from stressful experiences. Increased stresses in adolescence can cause cortisol levels to rise, which can affect teens' ability to function calmly and reasonably.

So, while teen bodies are a bundle of changes, the good news is that eventually your body adjusts, and the "raging" hormones calm down as you move into adulthood.

(Source: "Brain Development: The Teen Brain," National Institute on Drug Abuse (NIDA) for Teens.)

The Changing Brain And Behavior In Teens

One interpretation of all these findings is that in teens, the parts of the brain involved in emotional responses are fully online, or even more active than in adults, while the parts of the brain involved in keeping emotional, impulsive responses in check are still reaching maturity.

Such a changing balance might provide clues to a youthful appetite for novelty, and a tendency to act on impulse—without regard for risk.

While much is being learned about the teen brain, it is not yet possible to know to what extent a particular behavior or ability is the result of a feature of brain structure—or a change in brain structure. Changes in the brain take place in the context of many other factors, among them, inborn traits, personal history, family, friends, community, and culture.

What's Happening In Your Head?

No one feels good all the time. Teens are particularly vulnerable to a roller coaster of emotions because of major brain changes taking place between the ages of 12 and 25. These emotional ups and downs are all part of normal teen development.

But for teens suffering from mental health issues such as anxiety, depression, or ADHD, the stresses—from peers, family, or problems in school—may be more than they can handle. Some may start using drugs or alcohol as a way to cope, or to escape from anger, hurt, or disappointment. However, over time, these behaviors can lead to a bigger problem…addiction.

(Source: "Brain Development: The Teen Brain," National Institute on Drug Abuse (NIDA) for Teens.)

Teens And The Brain: More Questions For Research

Scientists continue to investigate the development of the brain and the relationship between the changes taking place, behavior, and health. The following questions are among the important ones that are targets of research:

- How do experience and environment interact with genetic preprogramming to shape the maturing brain, and as a result, future abilities and behavior? In other words, to what extent does what a teen does and learns shape his or her brain over the rest of a lifetime?

- In what ways do features unique to the teen brain play a role in the high rates of illicit substance use and alcohol abuse in the late teen to young adult years? Does the adolescent capacity for learning make this a stage of particular vulnerability to addiction?

- Why is it so often the case that, for many mental disorders, symptoms first emerge during adolescence and young adulthood?

This last question has been the central reason to study brain development from infancy to adulthood. Scientists increasingly view mental illnesses as developmental disorders that have their roots in the processes involved in how the brain matures. By studying how the circuitry of the brain develops, scientists hope to identify when and for what reasons development goes off track. Brain imaging studies have revealed distinctive variations in growth patterns of brain tissue in youth who show signs of conditions affecting mental health. Ongoing research is providing information on how genetic factors increase or reduce vulnerability to mental illness; and how experiences during infancy, childhood, and adolescence can increase the risk of mental illness or protect against it.

The Adolescent And Adult Brain

It is not surprising that the behavior of adolescents would be a study in change, since the brain itself is changing in such striking ways. Scientists emphasize that the fact that the teen brain is in transition doesn't mean it is somehow not up to par. It is different from both a child's and an adult's in ways that may equip youth to make the transition from dependence to independence. The capacity for learning at this age, an expanding social life, and a taste for exploration and limit testing may all, to some extent, be reflections of age-related biology.

Understanding the changes taking place in the brain at this age presents an opportunity to intervene early in mental illnesses that have their onset at this age. Research findings on the brain may also serve to help adults understand the importance of creating an environment in which teens can explore and experiment while helping them avoid behavior that is destructive to themselves and others.

Alcohol And The Teen Brain

Adults drink more frequently than teens, but when teens drink they tend to drink larger quantities than adults. There is evidence to suggest that the adolescent brain responds to alcohol differently than the adult brain, perhaps helping to explain the elevated risk of binge drinking in youth. Drinking in youth, and intense drinking are both risk factors for later alcohol dependence. Findings on the developing brain should help clarify the role of the changing brain in youthful drinking, and the relationship between youth drinking and the risk of addiction later in life.

The Teen Brain: Six Things To Know

Did you know that big and important changes are happening to the brain during adolescence? Here are six things to know about the teen brain:

1. **Your brain does not keep getting bigger as you get older**

   For girls, the brain reaches its largest physical size around 11 years old and for boys, the brain reaches its largest physical size around age 14. Of course, this difference in age does not mean either boys or girls are smarter than one another!

2. **But that doesn't mean your brain is done maturing**

For both boys and girls, although your brain may be as large as it will ever be, your brain doesn't finish developing and maturing until your mid- to late-20s. The front part of the brain, called the prefrontal cortex, is one of the last brain regions to mature. It is the area responsible for planning, prioritizing and controlling impulses.

3. **The teen brain is ready to learn and adapt**

In a digital world that is constantly changing, the adolescent brain is well prepared to adapt to new technology—and is shaped in return by experience.

4. **Many mental disorders appear during adolescence**

All the big changes the brain is experiencing may explain why adolescence is the time when many mental disorders—such as schizophrenia, anxiety, depression, bipolar disorder, and eating disorders—emerge.

5. **The teen brain is resilient**

Although adolescence is a vulnerable time for the brain and for teenagers in general, most teens go on to become healthy adults. Some changes in the brain during this important phase of development actually may help protect against long-term mental disorders.

6. **Teens need more sleep than children and adults**

Although it may seem like teens are lazy, science shows that melatonin levels (or the "sleep hormone" levels) in the blood naturally rise later at night and fall later in the morning than in most children and adults. This may explain why many teens stay up late and struggle with getting up in the morning. Teens should get about 9–10 hours of sleep a night, but most teens don't get enough sleep. A lack of sleep makes paying attention hard, increases impulsivity and may also increase irritability and depression.

Chapter 3

Why Is Mental Health Important?

Your mental health is very important. You will not have a healthy body if you don't also take care of your mind. People depend on you. It's important for you to take care of yourself so that you can do the important things in life—whether it's working, learning, taking care of your family, volunteering, enjoying the outdoors, or whatever is important to you.

Good mental health helps you enjoy life and cope with problems. It offers a feeling of well-being and inner strength. Just as you take care of your body by eating right and exercising, you can do things to protect your mental health. In fact, eating right and exercising can help maintain good mental health. You don't automatically have good mental health just because you don't have mental health illness. You have to work to keep your mind healthy.

Mental Health Awareness

Mental health is critical for personal well-being at every stage of life. Mental disorders are real, disabling health conditions that have an immense impact on individuals and families in the United States and internationally. Mental disorders vary widely in type and severity. About one in four adults in the United States suffer from a diagnosable mental disorder in a given year. Depression is the leading cause of disability in the United States for individuals ages 15–44.

Two-thirds of people with diagnosable mental disorders do not seek treatment. Treatment is individualized and may include counseling, psychotherapy, medication therapy, rehabilitation, and attention to other mental and psychosocial problems. Research findings in genetics and neuroscience are providing important new insights and approaches for more effective interventions.

(Source: "Mental Health Awareness," Centers for Disease Control and Prevention (CDC).)

About This Chapter: This chapter includes text excerpted from "Good Mental Health," Office on Women's Health (OWH), U.S. Department of Health and Human Services (HHS), May 13, 2017.

Nutrition And Mental Health

The food you eat can have a direct effect on your energy level, physical health, and mood. A "healthy diet" is one that has enough of each essential nutrient, contains many foods from all of the basic food groups, provides the right amount of calories to maintain a healthy weight, and does not have too much fat, sugar, salt, or alcohol.

By choosing foods that can give you steady energy, you can help your body stay healthy. This may also help your mind feel good. The same diet doesn't work for every person. In order to find the best foods that are right for you, talk to your healthcare professional.

Some vitamins and minerals may help with the symptoms of depression. Experts are looking into how a lack of some nutrients—including folate, vitamin B12, calcium, iron, selenium, zinc, and omega-3—may contribute to depression in new mothers. Ask your doctor or another healthcare professional for more information.

Exercise And Mental Health

Regular physical activity is important to the physical and mental health of almost everyone, including older adults. Being physically active can help you continue to do the things you enjoy and stay independent as you age. Regular physical activity over long periods of time can produce long-term health benefits. That's why health experts say that everyone should be active every day to maintain their health.

If you are diagnosed with depression or anxiety, your doctor may tell you to exercise in addition to taking any medications or receiving counseling. This is because exercise has been shown to help with the symptoms of depression and anxiety. Your body makes certain chemicals, called endorphins, before and after you work out. They relieve stress and improve your mood. Exercise can also slow or stop weight gain, which is a common side effect of some medications used to treat mental health disorders.

Sleep And Mental Health

Your mind and body will feel better if you sleep well. Your body needs time every day to rest and heal. If you often have trouble sleeping—either falling asleep, or waking during the night and being unable to get back to sleep—one or several of the following ideas might be helpful to you:

- Go to bed at the same time every night and get up at the same time every morning. Avoid "sleeping in" (sleeping much later than your usual time for getting up). It will make you feel worse.

- Establish a bedtime "ritual" by doing the same things every night for an hour or two before bedtime so your body knows when it is time to go to sleep.

- Avoid caffeine, nicotine, and alcohol.

- Eat on a regular schedule and avoid a heavy meal prior to going to bed. Don't skip any meals.

- Eat plenty of dairy foods and dark green leafy vegetables.

- Exercise daily, but avoid strenuous or invigorating activity before going to bed.

- Play soothing music on a tape or CD that shuts off automatically after you are in bed.

- Try a turkey sandwich and a glass of milk before bedtime to make you feel drowsy.

- Try having a small snack before you go to bed, something like a piece of fruit and a piece of cheese, so you don't wake up hungry in the middle of the night. Have a similar small snack if you awaken in the middle of the night.

- Take a warm bath or shower before going to bed.

- Place a drop of lavender oil on your pillow.

- Drink a cup of herbal chamomile tea before going to bed.

You need to see your doctor if:

- You often have difficulty sleeping and the solutions listed above are not working for you

- You awaken during the night gasping for breath

- Your partner says that your breathing stops when you are sleeping

- You snore loudly

- You wake up feeling like you haven't been asleep

- You fall asleep often during the day

Stress And Mental Health

Stress can happen for many reasons. Stress can be brought about by a traumatic accident, death, or emergency situation. Stress can also be a side effect of a serious illness or disease.

There is also stress associated with daily life, the workplace, and family responsibilities. It's hard to stay calm and relaxed in our hectic lives. As women, we have many roles: spouse, mother, caregiver, friend, and/or worker. With all we have going on in our lives, it seems almost impossible to find ways to de-stress. But it's important to find those ways. Your health depends on it.

Common symptoms include:

- Headache

- Sleep disorders

- Difficulty concentrating

- Short-temper

- Upset stomach

- Job dissatisfaction

- Low morale

- Depression

- Anxiety

Remember to always make time for you. It's important to care for yourself. Think of this as an order from your doctor, so you don't feel guilty! No matter how busy you are, you can try to set aside at least 15 minutes each day in your schedule to do something for yourself, like taking a bubble bath, going for a walk, or calling a friend.

Chapter 4

Resilience: A Vital Component Of Mental Health

"Resilient" adolescents are those who have managed to cope effectively, even in the face of stress and other difficult circumstances, and are poised to enter adulthood with a good chance of positive mental health. A number of factors promote resilience in adolescents—among the most important are caring relationships with adults and an easy-going disposition. Adolescents themselves can use a number of strategies, including exercising regularly, to reduce stress and promote resilience. Schools and communities are also recognizing the importance of resilience and general "emotional intelligence" in adolescents' lives—a growing number of courses and community programs focus on adolescents' social-emotional learning and coping skills.

What Is Individual Resilience?

Individual resilience involves behaviors, thoughts, and actions that promote personal well-being and mental health. People can develop the ability to withstand, adapt to, and recover from stress and adversity—and maintain or return to a state of mental health wellbeing—by using effective coping strategies. We call this individual resilience.

A disaster can impair resilience due to stress, traumatic exposure, distressing psychological reactions, and disrupted social networks. Feelings of grief, sadness, and a range of other emotions are common after traumatic events. Resilient individuals, however, are able to work through the emotions and effects of stress and painful events and rebuild their lives.

About This Chapter: Text in this chapter begins with excerpts from "Positive Adolescent Mental Health: Resilience," U.S. Department of Health and Human Services (HHS), October 28, 2016; Text beginning with the heading "What Is Individual Resilience?" is excerpted from "Individual Resilience," Office of the Assistant Secretary for Preparedness and Response (ASPR), U.S. Department of Health and Human Services (HHS), June 8, 2015.

Resilience refers to an individual's ability to cope with adversity and adapt to challenges or change. Resilience develops over time and gives an individual the capacity not only to cope with life's challenges but also to be better prepared for the next stressful situation. Optimism and the ability to remain hopeful are essential to resilience and the process of recovery.

(Source: "Recovery And Recovery Support," Substance Abuse and Mental Health Services Administration (SAMHSA).)

What Contributes To Individual Resilience?

People develop resilience by learning better skills and strategies for managing stress and better ways of thinking about life's challenges. To be resilient one must tap into personal strengths and the support of family, friends, neighbors, and/or faith communities.

What Are The Characteristics That Support Individual Resilience?

Age, gender, health, biology, education level, cultural beliefs and traditions, and economic resources can play important roles in psychological resilience. The following characteristics also contribute to individual resilience:

- **Social support and close relationships with family and friends:** People who have close social support and strong connections with family and friends are able to get help during tough times and also enjoy their relationships during everyday life.

- **The ability to manage strong feelings and impulses:** People who are able to manage strong emotions are less likely to get overwhelmed, frustrated, or aggressive. People who are able to manage feelings can still feel sadness or loss, but they are also able to find healthy ways to cope and heal.

- **Good problem-solving skills:** People problem-solve daily. Thinking, planning, and solving problems in an organized way are important skills. Problem solving skills contribute to feelings of independence and self-competence.

- **Feeling in control:** After the chaos of a disaster, it can be useful to engage in activities that help people regain a sense of control. This will help support the healing and recovery process.

- **Asking for help and seeking resources:** Resourceful people will get needed help more quickly if they know how to ask questions, are creative in their thinking about situations, are good problem solvers and communicators, and have a good social network to reach out to.

- **Seeing yourself as resilient:** After a disaster many people may feel helpless and powerless, especially when there has been vast damage to the community. Being able to see yourself as resilient, rather than as helpless or as a victim, can help build psychological resilience.

- **Coping with stress in healthy ways:** People get feelings of pleasure and self-worth from doing things well. Strategies that use positive and meaningful ways to cope are better than those which can be harmful such as drinking too much or smoking.

- **Helping others and finding positive meaning in life:** Positive emotions like gratitude, joy, kindness, love, and contentment can come from helping others. Acts of generosity can add meaning and purpose to your life, even in the face of tragedy.

Resilient individuals are able to:

- Care for themselves and others day-to-day and during emergency situations.

- Actively support their neighborhoods, workplaces, and communities to recover after disaster.

- Be confident and hopeful about overcoming present and future difficulties.

- Get needed resources more effectively and quickly.

- Be physically and mentally healthier and have overall lower recovery expenses and service needs.

- Miss fewer days of work.

- Maintain stable family and social connections.

- Re-establish routines more quickly, which helps children and adults alike.

Ways To Strengthen Resilience

You can build your resilience by taking care of your health, managing stress, and being an active participant in the life of your community. For example, try to:

- Develop coping skills and practice stress management activities, such as yoga, exercise, and meditation.

- Eat healthy and exercise.

- Get plenty of sleep.

- Maintain social connections to people and groups that are meaningful for you.

- Volunteer in your community.

- Get training in First Aid, Cardiopulmonary resuscitation (CPR), Community emergency response team (CERT), and Psychological First Aid.

- Create evacuation and family reunification plans.

- Make a disaster kit and stock supplies to shelter in place for up to 3 days.

- Find things that bring you pleasure and enjoyment such as reading a book or watching a movie, writing in a journal, or engaging in an art activity.

Does Individual Resilience Help Build Community Resilience?

Yes! Individual resilience is important to community resilience in that healthy people make for a healthier community. Healthy communities are better able to manage and recover from disasters and other emergencies.

Chapter 5

Defining Mental Illness

Mental Health Basics

The term mental health is commonly used in reference to mental illness. However, knowledge in the field has progressed to a level that appropriately differentiates the two. Although mental health and mental illness are related, they represent different psychological states

Mental health is "a state of well-being in which the individual realizes his or her own abilities, can cope with the normal stresses of life, can work productively and fruitfully, and is able to make a contribution to his or her community." It is estimated that only about 17 percent of U.S. adults are considered to be in a state of optimal mental health. There is emerging evidence that positive mental health is associated with improved health outcomes.

Mental illness is defined as "collectively all diagnosable mental disorders" or "health conditions that are characterized by alterations in thinking, mood, or behavior (or some combination thereof) associated with distress and/or impaired functioning." Depression is the most common type of mental illness, affecting more than 26 percent of the U.S. adult population. It has been estimated that by the year 2020, depression will be the second leading cause of disability throughout the world, trailing only ischemic heart disease.

About This Chapter: Text beginning with the heading "Mental Health Basics" is excerpted from "Mental Health Basics," Centers for Disease Control and Prevention (CDC), July 1, 2011. Reviewed July 2017; Text under the heading "Mental Illnesses" is excerpted from "Mental Illness," Centers for Disease Control and Prevention (CDC), August 11, 2016; Text beginning with the heading "Child And Adolescent Mental Health" is excerpted from "Child And Adolescent Mental Health," National Institute of Mental Health (NIMH), April 2017; Text under the heading "Stigma And Mental Illness" is excerpted from "Stigma And Mental Illness," Centers for Disease Control and Prevention (CDC), June 18, 2015. Text under the heading "Mental Health Treatment Options" is excerpted from "Mental Health—Treatment Options," Youth.gov, October 5, 2012. Reviewed July 2017.

Evidence has shown that mental disorders, especially depressive disorders, are strongly related to the occurrence, successful treatment, and course of many chronic diseases including diabetes, cancer, cardiovascular disease, asthma, and obesity and many risk behaviors for chronic disease; such as, physical inactivity, smoking, excessive drinking, and insufficient sleep.

Mental Health Indicators

In the healthcare and public health arena, more emphasis and resources have been devoted to screening, diagnosis, and treatment of mental illness than mental health. Little has been done to protect the mental health of those free of mental illness. Researchers suggest that there are indicators of mental health, representing three domains. These include the following:

- Emotional well-being

  - such as perceived life satisfaction, happiness, cheerfulness, peacefulness.

- Psychological well-being

  - such as self-acceptance, personal growth including openness to new experiences, optimism, hopefulness, purpose in life, control of one's environment, spirituality, self-direction, and positive relationships.

- Social well-being

  - social acceptance, beliefs in the potential of people and society as a whole, personal self-worth and usefulness to society, sense of community.

The former surgeon general notes that there are social determinants of mental health as there are social determinants of general health that need to be in place to support mental health. These include adequate housing, safe neighborhoods, equitable jobs and wages, quality education, and equity in access to quality healthcare.

Mental Illnesses

Mental illnesses refer to disorders generally characterized by dysregulation of mood, thought, and/or behavior, as recognized by the *Diagnostic and Statistical Manual, 4th edition,* of the American Psychiatric Association (DSM-IV). Mood disorders are among the most pervasive of all mental disorders and include major depression, in which the individual commonly reports feeling, for a time period of two weeks or more, sad or blue, uninterested in things previously of interest, psychomotor retardation or agitation, and increased or decreased appetite since the depressive episode ensued.

Depression

Depression is a serious medical illness and an important public health issue. Depression is characterized by persistent sadness and sometimes irritability (particularly in children) and is one of the leading causes of disease or injury worldwide for both men and women. Depression can cause suffering for depressed individuals and can also have negative effects on their families and the communities in which they live. The economic burden of depression, including workplace costs, direct costs and suicide-related costs, was estimated to be $210.5 billion in 2010.

Depression is associated with significant healthcare needs, school problems, loss of work, and earlier mortality.

Depression—

- Is associated with an increased risk for mortality from suicide as well as other causes, such as heart disease

- Is associated with lower workplace productivity and more absenteeism, which result in lower income and higher unemployment.

- Is associated with higher risk for other conditions and behaviors, including:

  - Other mental disorders (anxiety disorders, substance use disorders, eating disorders)

  - Smoking

Although effective treatments are available, many individuals with depression do not have access to treatment or do not take advantage of services. If not effectively treated, depression is likely to become a chronic disease. Just experiencing one episode of depression places an individual at a 50 percent risk for experiencing another episode, and further increases the chances of having more depression episodes in the future.

Public health surveillance systems measure the prevalence and impact of depression providing valuable information that can be used to guide mental health promotion, mental illness prevention, and treatment programs.

Anxiety

Anxiety disorders are characterized by excessive and unrealistic worry about everyday tasks or events, or may be specific to certain objects or rituals. Simple phobias involve excessive anxiety evoked by specific objects (e.g., marked fear of snakes). As its name implies, social phobias are fears of interacting with others, particularly in large groups. In obsessive-compulsive disorder (OCD), the individual experiences an obsession—an intrusive and recurrent thought, idea, sensation or feeling—coupled with a compulsion—a behavior that is recurrent and ritualized, such as checking, avoiding, or counting. In addition to being helped by pharmacotherapies, anxiety disorders are often addressed by exposure (to the object or event obsessed over) and response prevention—not permitting the compulsive behavior, to help the individual learn that it is not needed.

Psychotic Disorders

Psychotic disorders are characterized by dysregulation of thought processes. In particular, schizophrenia has hallmark symptoms of delusions—which are false beliefs—and hallucinations—which are hearing and/or seeing sensory information which is not actually present and is not apparent to others. Schizoaffective disorder is a disorder in which, as its name implies, individuals have features of both schizophrenia and mood disorders. Typically, psychotic disorders are treated with antipsychotic medications and some forms of psychosocial interventions.

Bipolar Disorder

Bipolar disorder (formerly known as "manic-depressive disorder") is another major mood disorder in which the individual most commonly experiences episodes of depression and episodes of mania. Mania is characterized by clearly elevated, unrestrained, or irritable mood which may manifest in an exaggerated assessment of self-importance or grandiosity, sleeplessness, racing thoughts, pressured speech, and the tendency to engage in activities which appear pleasurable, but have a high potential for adverse consequences. As is true for depression, medications and some forms of psychotherapy are effective in the treatment of bipolar disorder.

Child And Adolescent Mental Health

Mental health conditions and disorders don't only affect adults. Children and teens can experience mental health problems too. In fact, research has now shown that most mental disorders follow a developmental course that typically starts early in life. This is true not only of conditions such as autism and attention deficit hyperactivity disorder (ADHD), which are well known for having onset in childhood, but also for mood, anxiety, and psychotic disorders. So, many people who suffer from depression, social phobia, obsessive-compulsive disorder, bipolar disorder, or schizophrenia showed signs before they were 24 years old.

Like adults, children and teens can sometimes experience intense emotions as they get older or go through stressful or traumatic events in their lives. For example, it is common for children to feel anxious about school or friendships, or for teens to have short periods of depression after a death in the family.

Mental disorders are different. They can cause ongoing, severe symptoms that affect how a child feels, thinks, acts, and handles daily activities, such as going to school, sleeping, or eating. It is important to know the signs and seek help if needed.

Mental Illness Warning Signs

It can be tough to tell if troubling behavior in a child is just part of growing up or a problem that should be discussed with a health professional. But if there are signs and symptoms that last weeks or months; and if these issues interfere with the child's daily life, not only at home but at school and with friends, you should contact a health professional.

Your child or teen might need help if he or she:

- Often feels anxious or worried

- Has very frequent tantrums or is intensely irritable much of the time

- Has frequent stomachaches or headaches with no physical explanation

- Is in constant motion, can't sit quietly for any length of time

- Has trouble sleeping, including frequent nightmares

- Loses interest in things he or she used to enjoy

- Avoids spending time with friends

- Has trouble doing well in school, or grades decline

- Fears gaining weight; exercises, diets obsessively

- Has low or no energy

- Has spells of intense, inexhaustible activity

- Harms herself/himself, such as cutting or burning her/his skin

- Engages in risky, destructive behavior

- Harms self or others

- Smokes, drinks, or uses drugs

- Has thoughts of suicide

- Thinks his or her mind is controlled or out of control, hears voices

Mental illnesses can be treated. If you are a child or teen, talk to your parents, school counselor, or healthcare provider. If you are unsure where to go for help, ask your pediatrician or family doctor.

It may be helpful for children and teens to save several emergency numbers to their cell phones. The ability to get immediate help for themselves or for a friend can make a difference.

- The phone number for a trusted friend or relative

- The nonemergency number for the local police department

- The Crisis Text Line: 741741

- The National Suicide Prevention Lifeline: 1-800-273-TALK (1-800-273-8255)

> Many mental illnesses affect both men and women however men may be less likely to talk about their feelings and seek help. Recognizing the signs that someone may have a mood or mental disorder is the first step toward getting treatment and living a better life.
>
> Men and women experience many of the same mental disorders but their willingness to talk about their feelings may be very different. This is one of the reasons that their symptoms may be very different as well. For example, some men with depression or an anxiety disorder hide their emotions and may appear to be angry or aggressive while many women will express sadness. Some men may turn to drugs or alcohol to try to cope with their emotional issues. Sometimes mental health symptoms appear to be physical issues. For example, a racing heart, tightening chest, ongoing headaches, and digestive issues can be a sign of an emotional problem.
>
> *(Source: "Men And Mental Health," National Institute of Mental Health (NIMH).)*

Stigma And Mental Illness

Stigma has been defined as an attribute that is deeply discrediting. This stigmatized trait sets the bearer apart from the rest of society, bringing with it feelings of shame and isolation. Often, when a person with a stigmatized trait is unable to perform an action because of the condition, other people view the person as the problem rather than viewing the condition as the problem. More recent definitions of stigma focus on the results of stigma—the prejudice, avoidance, rejection and discrimination directed at people believed to have an illness, disorder or other trait perceived to be undesirable. Stigma causes needless suffering, potentially causing a person to deny symptoms, delay treatment and refrain from daily activities. Stigma can exclude people from access to housing, employment, insurance, and appropriate medical care.

Thus, stigma can interfere with prevention efforts, and examining and combating stigma is a public health priority.

The Substance Abuse and Mental Health Services Administration (SAMHSA) and the Centers for Disease Control and Prevention (CDC) have examined public attitudes toward mental illness in two surveys. In a survey, only one-quarter of young adults between the ages of 18–24 believed that a person with mental illness can eventually recover. Adults in 37 states and territories were surveyed about their attitudes toward mental illness, using the Behavioral Risk Factor Surveillance System Mental Illness and Stigma module. This study found that:

- 78 percent of adults with mental health symptoms and 89 percent of adults without such symptoms agreed that treatment can help persons with mental illness lead normal lives.

- 57 percent of adults without mental health symptoms believed that people are caring and sympathetic to persons with mental illness.

- Only 25 percent of adults with mental health symptoms believed that people are caring and sympathetic to persons with mental illness.

These findings highlight both the need to educate the public about how to support persons with mental illness and the need to reduce barriers for those seeking or receiving treatment for mental illness.

Mental Health Treatment Options

Mental health treatment can includes a variety of different approaches and occur in a variety of settings. Services provided depend on the needs and choices of the youth and his or her family, and the diagnosis and severity of the problem. They may consist of services such as psychotherapy with an evidence-based practice, peer mentoring, care coordination, medication, or a combination of all approaches.

In the United States, 75 to 80 percent of children and youth in need of mental health services do not receive them. This can be for a variety of reasons, including:

- discrimination and negative attitudes attached to seeking help for mental health issues,
- cultural beliefs and practices,
- access to services/supports,
- availability of providers,

- not knowing where to start, or

- confusion about who to see and what advice to take.

Youth may be receiving services in specialty treatment centers, educational settings, general medical settings, or a combination of settings. In 2008,

- 12.7 percent of youths aged 12 to 17 received treatment or counseling for problems with behavior or emotions in a specialty mental health setting (inpatient or outpatient care);

- 11.8 percent of youths received services in an education setting;

- 2.9 percent received mental health services in a general medical setting in the past 12 months; and

- 5.3 percent of youth received mental health services from both a specialty setting and either an education or a general medical setting (i.e., care from multiple settings).

Chapter 6

Causes And Warning Signs Of Mental Illness

Like adults, children and adolescents can have mental health or substance use problems that interfere with the way they think, feel, and act. Such problems—if not addressed—may interfere with learning and the ability to form and sustain friendships, contribute to disciplinary problems and family conflicts, and increase risky behaviors.

Mental Health Problem Common In Young People

Serious mental health problems often are a factor in drug abuse and suicide. Mental health and substance use problems are common in young people. Almost 21 percent of U.S. children and adolescents have a diagnosable mental health or addictive disorder that affects their ability to function. In any given year, 5 percent to 9 percent of youths ages 9–17 have a serious emotional disturbance that causes substantial impairment in how they function at home, at school, or in the community. Adolescents face a greater risk than adults of developing drug or alcohol use problems; 7.6 percent of adolescents ages 12–17 have met the criteria for dependence on and/or abuse of illicit drugs or alcohol. Mental health problems in adolescents often increase their use of substances such as alcohol, marijuana, and other drugs.

> Young people experience some of the highest prevalence rates of mental illness and yet have some of the lowest help seeking rates of any group. Additionally, childhood emotional and behavioral disorders are the most costly of all illnesses in children and youth.

About This Chapter: This chapter includes text excerpted from "Identifying Mental Health And Substance Use Problems Of Children And Adolescents: A Guide For Child-Serving Organizations," Substance Abuse and Mental Health Services Administration (SAMHSA), 2012. Reviewed July 2017.

Early life experiences are important in shaping an individual's life into adulthood and can impact how an individual learns and responds to stressful events.

- When young children are exposed to repeated traumatic experiences (e.g., child abuse, witnessing violence), they are at increased risk of developing mental health problems, substance abuse, and chronic health problems (like heart disease and diabetes).
- The negative impacts of these early experiences (sometimes referred to as "toxic stress") can be prevented or reversed when a child has a relationship with a supportive, responsive, and caring adult at an early age.
- Adverse Childhood Experiences, or ACEs, is a term that describes all types of abuse, neglect, and other traumatic experiences that occur to individuals under the age of 18. These can have a profound impact on that child's future health. In fact, a person who experiences four or more ACEs were 7.4 times more likely to consider themselves alcoholics, 3.9 times more likely to have chronic bronchitis or emphysema, 4.6 times more likely to report being depressed, and 1.9 times more likely to develop cancer

(Source: "Community Conversations About Mental Health," MentalHealth.gov, U.S. Department of Health and Human Services (HHS).)

Higher Risk Of Developing Mental Health

Some children and adolescents have a higher risk of developing mental health or substance use problems than others. Children and adolescents whose family members are living with conditions such as depression or other mental health disorders may have a higher risk of developing similar conditions. Youths with developmental disabilities and chronic medical conditions also can have a cooccurring mental health condition or can develop a substance use problem. For example, youths with asthma are at higher risk of developing depression than those who do not have asthma. Adolescents who are questioning their sexual identity or becoming aware of the possibility that they may be gay, lesbian, bisexual, or transgender can be at high risk for certain mental health disorders and misuse of substances. Children and adolescents in the juvenile justice system—especially girls—have been found to have a very high incidence of mental health and substance abuse disorders.

Factors That Can Influence The Risk Of Mental Health

Experiences and environments can increase or decrease the risk of mental health and substance use problems in children and adolescents. Protective factors such as family stability, supportive and nurturing relationships, a strong community, and faith organizations can help prevent certain kinds of problems from developing in children and adolescents. These protective factors also can be a source of support that helps children and adolescents cope with mental health and substance use problems if such problems develop.

Stress and psychological trauma are among a number of environmental risk factors that can contribute to the development of mental health or substance use problems in children and adolescents and also can increase the severity of such problems. Psychological trauma occurs when a youth experiences an intense event that threatens or causes harm to his or her emotional and physical well-being. A range of physiological and psychological behaviors can provide signs that the youth is having difficulty dealing with a traumatic event. However, these reactions are the body's normal response when confronted by danger. Some children and adolescents who have experienced a traumatic event will have longer lasting reactions that can interfere with their physical and emotional health, such as:

- Children and adolescents in families that have experienced significant losses may face greater challenges to healthy development than those without such losses.

- Children and adolescents from poor families have increased rates of developmental problems, stress, and uncertainty, which—along with other factors associated with poverty—can trigger behavioral health problems.

- Psychological trauma can trigger mental health and substance use problems. Children and adolescents who have been abused or neglected are at a higher risk of having mental health or substance use problems.

- Children and adolescents who were exposed to chronic violence at home or in their communities or who experienced a natural disaster or school violence are at heightened risk for mental health or substance use problems.

The Value Of Early Identification

Caregivers are usually the first to recognize early signs of problems in their children. Medical providers, teachers, or direct care workers in children's programs also are well positioned to improve the identification of mental health and substance use problems among the children and adolescents they serve. Just as schools screen for vision and hearing problems before such problems interfere with learning, service providers can develop early identification programs for mental health and substance use problems.

As children grow older, events in their lives may put them at risk for various problems. For children and adolescents who show clear signs of a mental health or substance use problem, a discrete identification process may not be necessary; instead, these youths can be referred directly for assessment.

Assessment

An assessment is conducted by a qualified, experienced mental health or substance abuse professional who gathers more information about the youth to determine whether an identified possible condition is, in fact, present. In addition to speaking with or observing the youth, the professional also should talk to parents or caregivers and—with the consent of parents or caregivers—to teachers or others who know the youth well. This step may involve determining whether a youth meets specific, defined criteria for a diagnosis according to a formal classification system in the *Diagnostic and Statistical Manual of Mental Disorders, 4th edition (DSM-IV) or the Diagnostic Classification of Mental Health and Developmental Disorders of Infancy and Early Childhood (DC:0-3R)*.

The professional also will collect information that is helpful in working with the child or adolescent and his or her family to develop a plan to address the problem. Because no screening or identification process is perfect, some children and adolescents may be incorrectly found to not have a mental health or substance use problem—when, in fact, they actually have one; or they incorrectly may be found to have a mental health or substance use problem when, in fact, they actually do not have one.

Intervention And/Or Treatment

The goal of identifying children and adolescents with a high likelihood of having mental health and substance use problems is to provide an appropriate intervention or to connect the youths and their families with assessment and treatment resources. Even when an organization can offer an intervention, it must be prepared for the possibility that a youth's problem may warrant additional, different, or more specialized services.

Methods To Identify Adolescents Who May Have Mental Illness

People who are not mental health or substance abuse professionals can employ two basic methods to identify children and adolescents who may have a mental health or substance use problem:

- Become familiar with signs of mental health and substance use problems.

- Administer a scientifically validated screening tool.

Become Familiar With Signs Of Mental Illness

Often, a child's or adolescent's behavior or appearance can provide signs of a mental health or substance use problem. These signs warrant action by caregivers and adults who work with the youth and can reliably identify the indicators so that the problem is assessed further and the child or adolescent has the opportunity to receive appropriate treatment. Materials are available to help educate adults about these signs.

Signs of some problems—such as depression, bulimia, or early stages of substance use— either may be actively concealed from adults or may not be readily apparent. Research has shown that these types of problems are difficult for caregivers and other adults to identify. The National Institute of Mental Health (NIMH) and the Substance Abuse and Mental Health Services Administration (SAMHSA) sponsored a research group of scientists and physicians to identify signs that indicate the need to take action and address mental health conditions in children and adolescents.

Higher risk populations can be identified in a number of ways, and common examples of their attributes are as follows:

- **Behavior or functioning.** Children and adolescents may demonstrate disciplinary problems; declining academic performance; or a marked change in behavior, mood, or functioning. However, some behavior signs are subtle and easily missed.

- **Illnesses or disabilities.** Children and adolescents with certain health problems are at higher risk for depression and other mental health problems. Children and adolescents serving as caretakers for ill or disabled parents or caregivers also are at high risk.

- **Environmental stress.** Children and adolescents living in a community with a high rate of poverty or violence are at increased risk of being identified with problems such as substance use or suicide, as compared to children and adolescents in other communities.

- **High-risk life situations.** Children and adolescents—particularly those who were prenatally exposed to drugs and alcohol—who come to the attention of child welfare systems or who are in homeless or domestic violence shelters are at high risk for mental health and substance use problems. Children or adolescents involved with the juvenile justice system also are associated with a much higher risk of mental health and substance use problems than children and adolescents in the general population.

- **Stressful events.** Stressful events or transitions that are the result of becoming homeless or entering into the child welfare system or juvenile detention involve significant losses and create considerable uncertainty for children and adolescents. Already vulnerable, these youths become even more so. State agencies and programs caring for these children and adolescents not only must safeguard the individual from harming himself or herself but also must ensure that the youth does not harm others. Screening for high-risk conditions as part of the intake process can help these agencies make initial placements and arrangements that are safe for the youth and others. Such screenings also assist in prioritizing assessments by a professional to address ongoing service and placement needs.

- **Traumatic events.** Children and adolescents not otherwise at risk may be exposed to an incident of violence or a natural disaster that warrants an effort to identify those who need assistance.

- **Age groups.** Certain ages or developmental stages might be prioritized for identification because of the high value of identifying problems or the low likelihood that problems will be identified elsewhere. For example, screening preschool children presents an early opportunity for intervention and has great value in preventing a problem or minimizing its impact on the child's future school performance and overall functioning. Screening teens in high school—a time when they no longer may see a primary care physician on a regular basis—has the potential to identify problems less likely to be identified elsewhere. Natural but stressful events associated with specific ages, such as the transition from elementary to middle school, also present potentially useful points of intervention.

- **Sexual orientation.** Children and adolescents questioning their sexual orientation or gender identity and those who identify as gay, lesbian, bisexual, transgender, queer, intersex, or two-spirit may have an elevated risk of mental health and substance use problems.

Administer A Scientifically Validated Screening Tool

The specific questions (items) included in a validated screening tool were tested on a large number of youths and were found to most accurately identify children and adolescents with a high likelihood of having mental health or substance use problems. Because different conditions are prone to arise at different stages of development or manifest differently at different ages, screening tools are designed for specific age ranges. Different tools or versions of a tool have been designed and tested to identify different conditions and to be answered by different informants. Informants can be physicians, parents or other caregivers, teachers, or other child service providers who are able to observe the youth; the informant also can be the child or adolescent if he or she is able to understand and answer the questions.

A number of studies have shown that such screening tools are better than the interviewing process used by primary care physicians or a clinical assessment conducted by mental health clinicians at identifying children and adolescents with mental health and substance use problems. The research results for the tested tools indicate the rate and type of problems found in different populations. Screening tools are the best brief method available for personnel who are not mental health or substance abuse professionals to identify children and adolescents at risk of mental health and substance use problems; but, like any medical test, no screening tool is correct all of the time.

Chapter 7

Mental Health Risk And Protective Factors

As youth grow and reach their developmental competencies, there are contextual variables that promote or hinder the process. These are frequently referred to as protective and risk factors.

The presence or absence and various combinations of protective and risk factors contribute to the mental health of youth. Identifying protective and risk factors in youth may guide the prevention and intervention strategies to pursue with them. Protective and risk factors may also influence the course mental health disorders might take if present.

A protective factor can be defined as "a characteristic at the biological, psychological, family, or community (including peers and culture) level that is associated with a lower likelihood of problem outcomes or that reduces the negative impact of a risk factor on problem outcomes." Conversely, a risk factor can be defined as "a characteristic at the biological, psychological, family, community, or cultural level that precedes and is associated with a higher likelihood of problem outcomes." Table 7.1 provides examples of protective and risk factors by five domains: youth, family, peer, community, and society.

Risk And Protective Factors Are Influential Over Time

Risk and protective factors can have influence throughout a person's entire lifespan. For example, risk factors such as poverty and family dysfunction can contribute to the development of mental and/or substance use disorders later in life. Risk and protective factors within

---

About This Chapter: This chapter includes text excerpted from "Risk And Protective Factors," Youth.gov, October 3, 2012. Reviewed July 2017.

one particular context—such as the family—may also influence or be influenced by factors in another context. Effective parenting has been shown to mediate the effects of multiple risk factors, including poverty, divorce, parental bereavement, and parental mental illness.

The more we understand how risk and protective factors interact, the better prepared we will be to develop appropriate interventions.

(Source: "Risk And Protective Factors," Substance Abuse and Mental Health Services Administration (SAMHSA).)

Table 7.1. Risk And Protective Factors For Mental, Emotional, And Behavioral Disorders In Adolescences

Risk Factors	Domains	Protective Factors
Depression	Individual	• Positive physical development
• Female gender		• Academic achievement/ intellectual development
• Early puberty		
• Difficult temperament: inflexibility, low positive mood, withdrawal, poor concentration		• High self-esteem
		• Emotional self-regulation
• Low self-esteem, perceived incompetence, negative explanatory and inferential style		• Good coping skills and problem-solving skills
• Anxiety		• Engagement and connections in two or more of the following contexts: school, with peers, in athletics, employment, religion, culture
• Low-level depressive symptoms and dysthymia		
• Insecure attachment		
• Poor social skills: communication and problem-solving skills		
• Extreme need for approval and social support		
Anxiety		
• Low self-esteem		
• Shyness		

Table 7.1. Continued

Risk Factors	Domains	Protective Factors
Substance Abuse • Emotional problems in childhood • Conduct disorder • Favorable attitudes toward drugs • Rebelliousness • Early substance use • Antisocial behavior		
Schizophrenia • Head injury • Marijuana use		
Conduct Disorder • Childhood exposure to lead or mercury (neurotoxins)		
Depression • Parental depression • Parent-child conflict • Poor parenting • Negative family environment (may include substance abuse in parents) • Child abuse/maltreatment • Single-parent family (for girls only) • Divorce • Marital conflict • Family conflict • Parent with anxiety	Family	• Family provides structure, limits, rules, monitoring, and predictability • Supportive relationships with family members • Clear expectations for behavior and values

Table 7.1. Continued

Risk Factors	Domains	Protective Factors
Anxiety • Parental/marital conflict • Family conflict (interactions between parents and children and among children) • Parental drug/alcohol use • Parental unemployment **Substance Abuse** • Substance use among parents • Lack of adult supervision • Poor attachment with parents **Schizophrenia** • Family dysfunction • Family member with schizophrenia **Conduct Disorder** • Poor parental supervision • Parental depression • Sexual abuse		
Depression • Peer rejection • Stressful events • Poor academic achievement • Poverty • Community-level stressful or traumatic events • School-level stressful or traumatic events • Community violence • School violence • Poverty • Traumatic event	School, Neighborhood, and Community	• Presence of mentors and support for development of skills and interests • Opportunities for engagement within school and community • Positive norms • Clear expectations for behavior • Physical and psychological safety

Table 7.1. Continued

Risk Factors	Domains	Protective Factors
Anxiety		
• School failure		
• Low commitment to school		
• Not college bound		
• Aggression toward peers		
• Associating with drug-using peers		
• Societal/community norms favor alcohol and drug use		
Schizophrenia		
• Urban setting		
• Poverty		
Conduct Disorder		
• Associating with deviant peers		
• Loss of close relationship or friends		

Chapter 8

Mental Health And Mental Disorders

Mental health is a state of successful performance of mental function, resulting in productive activities, fulfilling relationships with other people, and the ability to adapt to change and to cope with challenges. Mental health is essential to personal well-being, family and interpersonal relationships, and the ability to contribute to community or society.

Mental disorders are health conditions that are characterized by alterations in thinking, mood, and/or behavior that are associated with distress and/or impaired functioning. Mental disorders contribute to a host of problems that may include disability, pain, or death.

Mental illness is the term that refers collectively to all diagnosable mental disorders.

Mental Health In Adolescents

Important mental health habits—including coping, resilience, and good judgment—help adolescents to achieve overall wellbeing and set the stage for positive mental health in adulthood. Mood swings are common during adolescence. However, approximately one in five adolescents has a diagnosable mental disorder, such as depression and/or anxiety disorders. Friends and family can watch for warning signs of mental disorders and urge young people to get help. Effective treatments exist and may involve a combination of psychotherapy and medication. Unfortunately, less than half of adolescents with psychiatric disorders received any kind of treatment in the last year.

(Source: "Mental Health In Adolescents," Office of Adolescent Health (OAH), U.S. Department of Health and Human Services (HHS).)

About This Chapter: This chapter includes text excerpted from "Mental Health And Mental Disorders," Office of Disease Prevention and Health Promotion (ODPHP), U.S. Department of Health and Human Services (HHS), June 2, 2017.

Importance Of Mental Health

Mental disorders are among the most common causes of disability. The resulting disease burden of mental illness is among the highest of all diseases. In any given year, an estimated 18.1 percent (43.6 million) of U.S. adults ages 18 years or older suffered from any mental illness and 4.2 percent (9.8 million) suffered from a seriously debilitating mental illness. Neuropsychiatric disorders are the leading cause of disability in the United States, accounting for 18.7 percent of all years of life lost to disability and premature mortality. Moreover, suicide is the 10th leading cause of death in the United States, accounting for the deaths of approximately 43,000 Americans in 2014.

Mental health and physical health are closely connected. Mental health plays a major role in people's ability to maintain good physical health. Mental illnesses, such as depression and anxiety, affect people's ability to participate in health-promoting behaviors. In turn, problems with physical health, such as chronic diseases, can have a serious impact on mental health and decrease a person's ability to participate in treatment and recovery.

Understanding Mental Health And Mental Disorders

The existing model for understanding mental health and mental disorders emphasizes the interaction of social, environmental, and genetic factors throughout the lifespan. In behavioral health, researchers identify:

- Risk factors, which predispose individuals to mental illness

- Protective factors, which protect them from developing mental disorders

Researchers now know that the prevention of mental, emotional, and behavioral (MEB) disorders is inherently interdisciplinary and draws on a variety of different strategies.

Over the past 20 years, research on the prevention of mental disorders has progressed. The understanding of how the brain functions under normal conditions and in response to stressors, combined with knowledge of how the brain develops over time, has been essential to that progress. The major areas of progress include evidence that:

- MEB disorders are common and begin early in life

- The greatest opportunity for prevention is among young people

- There are multiyear effects of multiple preventive interventions on reducing substance abuse, conduct disorder, antisocial behavior, aggression, and child maltreatment

- The incidence of depression among pregnant women and adolescents can be reduced

- School-based violence prevention can reduce the base rate of aggressive problems in an average school by 25 to 33 percent

- There are potential indicated preventive interventions for schizophrenia

- Improving family functioning and positive parenting can have positive outcomes on mental health and can reduce poverty-related risk

- School-based preventive interventions aimed at improving social and emotional outcomes can also improve academic outcomes

- Interventions targeting families dealing with adversities, such as parental depression or divorce, can be effective in reducing risk for depression among children and increasing effective parenting

- Some preventive interventions have benefits that exceed costs, with the available evidence strongest for early childhood interventions

- Implementation is complex, and it is important that interventions be relevant to the target audiences

The progress identified above has led to a stronger understanding of the importance of protective factors. A Institute of Medicine (IOM) report advocates for multidisciplinary prevention strategies at the community level that support the development of children in healthy social environments. In addition to advancements in the prevention of mental disorders, there continues to be steady progress in treating mental disorders as new drugs and stronger evidence-based outcomes become available.

Emerging Issues In Mental Health And Mental Disorders

As the Federal Government begins to implement the health reform legislation, it will give attention to providing services for individuals with mental illness and substance use disorders, including new opportunities for access to and coverage for treatment and prevention services.

Part Two
Mood And Anxiety Disorders

Chapter 9

Depression

Depression Is A Real Illness

Sadness is something we all experience. It is a normal reaction to difficult times in life and usually passes with a little time.

When a person has depression, it interferes with daily life and normal functioning. It can cause pain for both the person with depression and those who care about him or her. Doctors call this condition "depressive disorder," or "clinical depression." It is a real illness. It is not a sign of a person's weakness or a character flaw. You can't "snap out of" clinical depression. Most people who experience depression need treatment to get better.

> You are not alone. There are ways you can feel better. If you have been feeling sad, hopeless, or irritable for what seems like a long time, you might have depression.
>
> - Depression is a real, treatable brain illness, or health problem.
> - Depression can be caused by big transitions in life, stress, or changes in your body's chemicals that affect your thoughts and moods.
> - Even if you feel hopeless, depression gets better with treatment.
> - There are lots of people who understand and want to help you.
> - Ask for help as early as you can so you can get back to being yourself.
>
> *(Source: "Teen Depression," National Institute of Mental Health (NIMH).)*

About This Chapter: This chapter includes text excerpted from "Depression: What You Need To Know," National Institute of Mental Health (NIMH), December 13, 2015.

Signs And Symptoms Of Depression

Sadness is only a small part of depression. Some people with depression may not feel sadness at all. Depression has many other symptoms, including physical ones. If you have been experiencing any of the following signs and symptoms for at least 2 weeks, you may be suffering from depression:

- Persistent sad, anxious, or "empty" mood

- Feelings of hopelessness, pessimism

- Feelings of guilt, worthlessness, helplessness

- Loss of interest or pleasure in hobbies and activities

- Decreased energy, fatigue, being "slowed down"

- Difficulty concentrating, remembering, making decisions

- Difficulty sleeping, early-morning awakening, or oversleeping

- Appetite and/or weight changes

- Thoughts of death or suicide, suicide attempts

- Restlessness, irritability

- Persistent physical symptoms

Factors That Play A Role In Depression

Many factors may play a role in depression, including genetics, brain biology and chemistry, and life events such as trauma, loss of a loved one, a difficult relationship, an early childhood experience, or any stressful situation.

Depression can happen at any age, but often begins in the teens or early 20s or 30s. Most chronic mood and anxiety disorders in adults begin as high levels of anxiety in children. In fact, high levels of anxiety as a child could mean a higher risk of depression as an adult.

Depression can cooccur with other serious medical illnesses such as diabetes, cancer, heart disease, and Parkinson disease. Depression can make these conditions worse and vice versa. Sometimes medications taken for these illnesses may cause side effects that contribute to depression. A doctor experienced in treating these complicated illnesses can help work out the best treatment strategy.

Types Of Depression

There are several types of depressive disorders.

- **Major depression:** Severe symptoms that interfere with the ability to work, sleep, study, eat, and enjoy life. An episode can occur only once in a person's lifetime, but more often, a person has several episodes.

- **Persistent depressive disorder:** A depressed mood that lasts for at least 2 years. A person diagnosed with persistent depressive disorder may have episodes of major depression along with periods of less severe symptoms, but symptoms must last for 2 years.

Some forms of depression are slightly different, or they may develop under unique circumstances. They include:

- **Psychotic depression,** which occurs when a person has severe depression plus some form of psychosis, such as having disturbing false beliefs or a break with reality (delusions), or hearing or seeing upsetting things that others cannot hear or see (hallucinations).

- **Postpartum depression,** which is much more serious than the "baby blues" that many women experience after giving birth, when hormonal and physical changes and the new responsibility of caring for a newborn can be overwhelming. It is estimated that 10 to 15 percent of women experience postpartum depression after giving birth.

- **Seasonal affective disorder (SAD),** which is characterized by the onset of depression during the winter months, when there is less natural sunlight. The depression generally lifts during spring and summer. SAD may be effectively treated with light therapy, but nearly half of those with SAD do not get better with light therapy alone. Antidepressant medication and psychotherapy can reduce SAD symptoms, either alone or in combination with light therapy.

- **Bipolar disorder** is different from depression. The reason it is included in this list is because someone with bipolar disorder experiences episodes of extreme low moods (depression). But a person with bipolar disorder also experiences extreme high moods (called "mania").

Depression Affects Children And Teen In Different Ways

Not everyone who is depressed experiences every symptom. Some people experience only a few symptoms. Some people have many. The severity and frequency of symptoms, and how long they last, will vary depending on the individual and his or her particular illness. Symptoms may also vary depending on the stage of the illness.

Children

Before puberty, girls and boys are equally likely to develop depression. A child with depression may pretend to be sick, refuse to go to school, cling to a parent, or worry that a parent may die. Because normal behaviors vary from one childhood stage to another, it can be difficult to tell whether a child is just going through a temporary "phase" or is suffering from depression. Sometimes the parents become worried about how the child's behavior has changed, or a teacher mentions that "your child doesn't seem to be himself." In such a case, if a visit to the child's pediatrician rules out physical symptoms, the doctor will probably suggest that the child be evaluated, preferably by a mental health professional who specializes in the treatment of children. Most chronic mood disorders, such as depression, begin as high levels of anxiety in children.

Teens

The teen years can be tough. Teens are forming an identity apart from their parents, grappling with gender issues and emerging sexuality, and making independent decisions for the first time in their lives. Occasional bad moods are to be expected, but depression is different.

Older children and teens with depression may sulk, get into trouble at school, be negative and irritable, and feel misunderstood. If you're unsure if an adolescent in your life is depressed or just "being a teenager," consider how long the symptoms have been present, how severe they are, and how different the teen is acting from his or her usual self. Teens with depression may also have other disorders such as anxiety, eating disorders, or substance abuse. They may also be at higher risk for suicide.

Children and teenagers usually rely on parents, teachers, or other caregivers to recognize their suffering and get them the treatment they need. Many teens don't know where to go for mental health treatment or believe that treatment won't help. Others don't get help because they think depression symptoms may be just part of the typical stress of school or being a teen. Some teens worry what other people will think if they seek mental healthcare.

Depression often persists, recurs, and continues into adulthood, especially if left untreated. If you suspect a child or teenager in your life is suffering from depression, speak up right away.

Tips for talking to a depressed child or teen:

- Offer emotional support, understanding, patience, and encouragement.

- Talk to your child, not necessarily about depression, and listen carefully.

- Never discount the feelings your child expresses, but point out realities and offer hope.

- Never ignore comments about suicide.

- Remind your child that with time and treatment, the depression will lift.

Treatment For Depression

Depression, even the most severe cases, can be treated. The earlier treatment begins, the more effective it is. Most adults see an improvement in their symptoms when treated with antidepressant drugs, talk therapy (psychotherapy), or a combination of both.

If you think you may have depression, start by making an appointment to see your doctor or healthcare provider. This could be your primary doctor or a health provider who specializes in diagnosing and treating mental health conditions (psychologist or psychiatrist). Certain medications, and some medical conditions, such as viruses or a thyroid disorder, can cause the same symptoms as depression. A doctor can rule out these possibilities by doing a physical exam, interview, and lab tests. If the doctor can find no medical condition that may be causing the depression, the next step is a psychological evaluation.

Talking To Your Doctor

How well you and your doctor talk to each other is one of the most important parts of getting good healthcare. But talking to your doctor isn't always easy. It takes time and effort on your part as well as your doctor's.

To prepare for your appointment, make a list of:

- Any symptoms you've had, including any that may seem unrelated to the reason for your appointment:

  - When did your symptoms start?

  - How severe are your symptoms?

- Have the symptoms occurred before?

- If the symptoms have occurred before, how were they treated?

- Key personal information, including any major stresses or recent life changes

- All medications, vitamins, or other supplements that you're taking, including how much and how often

- Questions to ask your health provider

If you don't have a primary doctor or are not at ease with the one you currently see, now may be the time to find a new doctor. Whether you just moved to a new city, changed insurance providers, or had a bad experience with your doctor or medical staff, it is worthwhile to spend time finding a doctor you can trust.

Tests and Diagnosis

Your doctor or healthcare provider will examine you and talk to you at the appointment. Your doctor may do a physical exam and ask questions about your health and symptoms. There are no lab tests that can specifically diagnose depression, but your doctor may also order some lab tests to rule out other conditions.

Ask questions if the doctor's explanations or instructions are unclear, bring up problems even if the doctor doesn't ask, and let the doctor know if you have concerns about a particular treatment or change in your daily life.

Your doctor may refer you to a mental health professional, such as a psychiatrist, psychologist, social worker, or mental health counselor, who should discuss with you any family history of depression or other mental disorder, and get a complete history of your symptoms. The mental health professional may also ask if you are using alcohol or drugs, and if you are thinking about death or suicide.

Treatment

Depression is treated with medicines, talk therapy (where a person talks with a trained professional about his or her thoughts and feelings; sometimes called "psychotherapy"), or a combination of the two. Remember: No two people are affected the same way by depression. There is no "one-size-fits-all" for treatment. It may take some trial and error to find the treatment that works best for you.

If You Think A Loved One May Have Depression

If you know someone who is depressed, it affects you too. The most important thing you can do is to help your friend or relative get a diagnosis and treatment. You may need to make an appointment and go with him or her to see the doctor. Encourage your loved one to stay in treatment or to seek different treatment options if no improvement occurs after 6 to 8 weeks.

To help your friend or relative:

- Offer emotional support, understanding, patience, and encouragement.

- Talk to him or her, and listen carefully.

- Never dismiss feelings, but point out realities and offer hope.

- Never ignore comments about suicide and report them to your loved one's therapist or doctor.

- Invite your loved one out for walks, outings, and other activities. Keep trying if he or she declines, but don't push him or her to take on too much too soon.

- Provide assistance in getting to doctors' appointments.

- Remind your loved one that with time and treatment, the depression will lift.

Caring for someone with depression is not easy. Someone with depression may need constant support for a long period of time. Make sure you leave time for yourself and your own needs. If you feel you need additional support, there are support groups for caregivers too.

Chapter 10

Premenstrual Syndrome And Premenstrual Dysphoric Disorder

What Is Premenstrual Syndrome (PMS)?

Premenstrual syndrome (PMS) is a group of symptoms linked to the menstrual cycle. PMS symptoms occur 1 to 2 weeks before your period (menstruation or monthly bleeding) starts. The symptoms usually go away after you start bleeding. PMS can affect menstruating women of any age and the effect is different for each woman. For some people, PMS is just a monthly bother. For others, it may be so severe that it makes it hard to even get through the day. PMS goes away when your monthly periods stop, such as when you get pregnant or go through menopause.

What Causes PMS?

The causes of PMS are not clear, but several factors may be involved. Changes in hormones during the menstrual cycle seem to be an important cause. These changing hormone levels may affect some women more than others. Chemical changes in the brain may also be involved. Stress and emotional problems, such as depression, do not seem to cause PMS, but they may make it worse. Some other possible causes include:

- Low levels of vitamins and minerals

- Eating a lot of salty foods, which may cause you to retain (keep) fluid

- Drinking alcohol and caffeine, which may alter your mood and energy level

---

About This Chapter: This chapter includes text excerpted from "Premenstrual Syndrome," Office on Women's Health (OWH), U.S. Department of Health and Human Services (HHS), December 23, 2014.

What Are The Symptoms Of PMS?

PMS often includes both physical and emotional symptoms, such as:

- Acne

- Swollen or tender breasts

- Feeling tired

- Trouble sleeping

- Upset stomach, bloating, constipation, or diarrhea

- Headache or backache

- Appetite changes or food cravings

- Joint or muscle pain

- Trouble with concentration or memory

- Tension, irritability, mood swings, or crying spells

- Anxiety or depression

Symptoms vary from woman to woman.

Premenstrual Mood Changes

Hormones can affect a woman's mood throughout her lifetime. Sometimes the impact on mood can affect a woman's quality of life. Many times the symptoms that result can be managed with medicine and/or therapy.

Once a young woman starts menstruating, she may begin to experience emotional changes around the time of her period. About 75 percent of women with regular period cycles report unpleasant physical or psychological symptoms before their periods. Premenstrual syndrome, or PMS, affects 30 to 80 percent of women.

Lifestyle changes may help make the symptoms of PMS and PMDD better. Some doctors suggest that women:

- Eat lesser amounts of caffeine, sugar, and sodium

- Drink less alcohol

- Don't smoke

- Get plenty of sleep

- Exercise more
- Try talk therapy

Medications or supplements prescribed by your doctor can also help PMS and PMDD. These may include:

- Calcium (1200 mg per day was shown to reduce PMS symptoms)
- Selective serotonin reuptake inhibitors (SSRIs)
- Hormonal treatments such as oral contraceptives

For all women, simple lifestyle changes in diet, exercise, and stress management are usually encouraged. These changes do not have risks and may help you.

(Source: "Mental Health—Menstruation, Menopause, And Mental Health," National Women's Health Information Center (NWHIC), Office on Women's Health (OWH).)

How Do I Know If I Have PMS?

Your doctor may diagnose PMS based on which symptoms you have, when they occur, and how much they affect your life. If you think you have PMS, keep track of which symptoms you have and how severe they are for a few months. Record your symptoms each day on a calendar or PMS symptom tracker. Take this form with you when you see your doctor about your PMS.

Your doctor will also want to make sure you don't have one of the following conditions that shares symptoms with PMS:

- Depression
- Anxiety
- Menopause
- Chronic fatigue syndrome (CFS)
- Irritable bowel syndrome (IBS)
- Problems with the endocrine system, which makes hormones

How Common Is PMS?

There's a wide range of estimates of how many women suffer from PMS. The American College of Obstetricians and Gynecologists (ACOG) estimates that at least 85 percent of menstruating women have at least 1 PMS symptom as part of their monthly cycle. Most of these women have fairly mild symptoms that don't need treatment. Others (about 3 to 8 percent) have a more severe form of PMS, called premenstrual dysphoric disorder (PMDD).

PMS occurs more often in women who:

- Are between their late 20s and early 40s

- Have at least 1 child

- Have a family history of depression

- Have a past medical history of either postpartum depression or a mood disorder

What Is The Treatment For PMS?

Many things have been tried to ease the symptoms of PMS. No treatment works for every woman. You may need to try different ones to see what works for you. Some treatment options include:

- Lifestyle changes

- Medications

- Alternative therapies

Lifestyle Changes

If your PMS isn't so bad that you need to see a doctor, some lifestyle changes may help you feel better. Below are some steps you can take that may help ease your symptoms.

- Exercise regularly. Each week, you should get:

  - Two hours and 30 minutes of moderate-intensity physical activity;

  - One hour and 15 minutes of vigorous-intensity aerobic physical activity; or

  - A combination of moderate and vigorous-intensity activity; and

  - Muscle-strengthening activities on 2 or more days.

- Eat healthy foods, such as fruits, vegetables, and whole grains.

- Avoid salt, sugary foods, caffeine, and alcohol, especially when you're having PMS symptoms.

- Get enough sleep. Try to get about 8 hours of sleep each night.

- Find healthy ways to cope with stress. Talk to your friends, exercise, or write in a journal. Some women also find yoga, massage, or relaxation therapy helpful.

- Don't smoke.

Medications

Over-the-counter pain relievers may help ease physical symptoms, such as cramps, headaches, backaches, and breast tenderness. These include:

- Ibuprofen (for instance, Advil, Motrin, Midol Cramp)

- Ketoprofen (for instance, Orudis KT)

- Naproxen (for instance, Aleve)

- Aspirin

  In more severe cases of PMS, prescription medicines may be used to ease symptoms. One approach has been to use drugs that stop ovulation, such as birth control pills. Women on the pill report fewer PMS symptoms, such as cramps and headaches, as well as lighter periods.

Researchers continue to search for new ways to treat PMS. To learn more about current PMS treatment studies, visit the clinicaltrials.gov website. Talk to your doctor about whether taking part in a clinical trial might be right for you.

Alternative Therapies

Certain vitamins and minerals have been found to help relieve some PMS symptoms. These include:

- Folic acid (400 micrograms)

- Calcium with vitamin D

- Magnesium (400 milligrams)

- Vitamin B-6 (50 to 100 mg)

- Vitamin E (400 international units)

Pregnant or nursing women need the same amount of calcium as other women of the same age.

Some women find their PMS symptoms relieved by taking supplements such as:

- Black cohosh

- Chasteberry

- Evening primrose oil

Talk with your doctor before taking any of these products. Many have not been proven to work and they may interact with other medicines you are taking.

What Is Premenstrual Dysphoric Disorder (PMDD)?

A brain chemical called serotonin may play a role in premenstrual dysphoric disorder (PMDD), a severe form of PMS. The main symptoms, which can be disabling, include:

- Feelings of sadness or despair, or even thoughts of suicide

- Feelings of tension or anxiety

- Panic attacks

- Mood swings or frequent crying

- Lasting irritability or anger that affects other people

- Lack of interest in daily activities and relationships

- Trouble thinking or focusing

- Tiredness or low energy

- Food cravings or binge eating

- Trouble sleeping

- Feeling out of control

- Physical symptoms, such as bloating, breast tenderness, headaches, and joint or muscle pain

You must have 5 or more of these symptoms to be diagnosed with PMDD. Symptoms occur during the week before your period and go away after bleeding starts. Making some lifestyle changes may help ease PMDD symptoms. Antidepressants called selective serotonin reuptake inhibitors (SSRIs) have also been shown to help some women with PMDD. These drugs change serotonin levels in the brain.

Chapter 11

Seasonal Affective Disorder

Seasonal affective disorder (SAD) is a type of depression that comes and goes with the seasons, typically starting in the late fall and early winter and going away during the spring and summer. Depressive episodes linked to the summer can occur, but are much less common than winter episodes of SAD.

Signs And Symptoms Of Seasonal Affective Disorder (SAD)

Seasonal affective disorder (SAD) is not considered as a separate disorder. It is a type of depression displaying a recurring seasonal pattern. To be diagnosed with SAD, people must meet full criteria for major depression coinciding with specific seasons (appearing in the winter or summer months) for at least 2 years. Seasonal depressions must be much more frequent than any nonseasonal depressions.

Symptoms Of Major Depression

- Feeling depressed most of the day, nearly every day

- Feeling hopeless or worthless

- Having low energy

- Losing interest in activities you once enjoyed

- Having problems with sleep

About This Chapter: This chapter includes text excerpted from "Seasonal Affective Disorder," National Institute of Mental Health (NIMH), March 2016.

- Experiencing changes in your appetite or weight
- Feeling sluggish or agitated
- Having difficulty concentrating
- Having frequent thoughts of death or suicide.

Symptoms of the winter pattern of SAD include:

- Having low energy
- Hypersomnia
- Overeating
- Weight gain
- Craving for carbohydrates
- Social withdrawal (feel like "hibernating")

Symptoms of the less frequently occurring summer SAD include:

- Poor appetite with associated weight loss
- Insomnia
- Agitation
- Restlessness
- Anxiety
- Episodes of violent behavior

Risk Factors That Increase The Risk Of SAD

Attributes that may increase your risk of SAD include:

- **Younger Age.** Younger adults have a higher risk of SAD than older adults. SAD has been reported even in children and teens.
- **Being female.** SAD is diagnosed four times more often in women than men.
- **Living far from the equator.** SAD is more frequent in people who live far north or south of the equator. For example, 1 percent of those who live in Florida and 9 percent of those who live in New England or Alaska suffer from SAD.
- **Family history.** People with a family history of other types of depression are more likely to develop SAD than people who do not have a family history of depression.

- **Having depression or bipolar disorder.** The symptoms of depression may worsen with the seasons if you have one of these conditions (but SAD is diagnosed only if seasonal depressions are the most common).

The causes of SAD are unknown, but research has found some biological clues:

- **People with SAD may have trouble regulating one of the key neurotransmitters involved in mood, serotonin.** One study found that people with SAD have 5 percent more serotonin transporter protein in winter months than summer months. Higher serotonin transporter protein leaves less serotonin available at the synapse because the function of the transporter is to recycle neurotransmitter back into the presynaptic neuron.

- **People with SAD may overproduce the hormone melatonin.** Darkness increases production of melatonin, which regulates sleep. As winter days become shorter, melatonin production increases, leaving people with SAD to feel sleepier and more lethargic, often with delayed circadian rhythms.

- **People with SAD also may produce less vitamin D.** Vitamin D is believed to play a role in serotonin activity. Vitamin D insufficiency may be associated with clinically significant depression symptoms.

Treatments And Therapies For SAD

There are four major types of treatment for SAD:

- Medication

- Light therapy

- Psychotherapy

- Vitamin D

These may be used alone or in combination.

Medication

Selective serotonin reuptake inhibitors (SSRIs) are used to treat SAD. The U.S. Food and Drug Administration (FDA) has also approved the use of bupropion, another type of antidepressant, for treating SAD.

As with other medications, there are side effects to SSRIs. Talk to your doctor about the possible risks of using this medication for your condition. You may need to try several different antidepressant medications before finding the one that improves your symptoms without causing problematic side effects.

Light Therapy

Light therapy has been a mainstay of treatment for SAD since the 1980s. The idea behind light therapy is to replace the diminished sunshine of the fall and winter months using daily exposure to bright, artificial light. Symptoms of SAD may be relieved by sitting in front of a light box first thing in the morning, on a daily basis from the early fall until spring. Most typically, light boxes filter out the ultraviolet rays and require 20–60 minutes of exposure to 10,000 lux of cool-white fluorescent light, an amount that is about 20 times greater than ordinary indoor lighting.

The cause of SAD is not well understood. It is believed that the decreasing daylight available in fall and winter triggers a depressive episode in people predisposed to develop the disorder. However, no studies have established a causal relationship between decreasing daylight and the development of winter SAD.

One of the most effective remedies for dealing with the condition is light therapy. Light therapy has proven effective in a limited number of small, placebo-controlled studies.

The usual dose is 10,000 lux (the intensity of light that hits or passes through a surface) beginning with one 10-to-15-minute session per day, usually in the morning, gradually increasing to 30 to 45 minutes per day, depending upon response.

It may take four-to-six weeks to see a response, although some patients improve within days. Therapy is continued until sufficient daily light exposure is available through other sources, typically from springtime sun.

Light therapy is considered first-line therapy in patients who are not severely suicidal, have medical reasons to avoid antidepressant drugs, have a history of a positive response to light therapy, or if the patient specifically requests it.

(Source: "Seasonal Affective Disorder," U.S. Department of Veterans Affairs (VA).)

Psychotherapy

Cognitive behavioral therapy (CBT) is type of psychotherapy that is effective for SAD. Traditional cognitive behavioral therapy has been adapted for use with SAD (CBT-SAD). CBT-SAD relies on basic techniques of CBT such as identifying negative thoughts and replacing them with more positive thoughts along with a technique called behavioral activation.

Behavioral activation seeks to help the person identify activities that are engaging and pleasurable, whether indoors or outdoors, to improve coping with winter.

Vitamin D

At present, vitamin D supplementation by itself is not regarded as an effective SAD treatment. The reason behind its use is that low blood levels of vitamin D were found in people with SAD. The low levels are usually due to insufficient dietary intake or insufficient exposure to sunshine. However, the evidence for its use has been mixed. While some studies suggest vitamin D supplementation may be as effective as light therapy, others found vitamin D had no effect.

Chapter 12

Bipolar Disorder

Does your child go through intense mood changes? Does your child have extreme behavior changes? Does your child get much more excited and active than other kids his or her age? Do other people say your child is too excited or too moody? Do you notice he or she has highs and lows much more often than other children? Do these mood changes affect how your child acts at school or at home?

Some children and teens with these symptoms may have bipolar disorder, a serious mental illness.

What Is Bipolar Disorder?

Bipolar disorder is a serious brain illness. It is also called manic-depressive illness or manic depression. Children with bipolar disorder go through unusual mood changes. Sometimes they feel very happy or "up," and are much more energetic and active than usual, or than other kids their age. This is called a manic episode. Sometimes children with bipolar disorder feel very sad and "down," and are much less active than usual. This is called depression or a depressive episode.

Bipolar disorder is not the same as the normal ups and downs every kid goes through. Bipolar symptoms are more powerful than that. The mood swings are more extreme and are accompanied by changes in sleep, energy level, and the ability to think clearly. Bipolar symptoms are so strong, they can make it hard for a child to do well in school or get along with friends and family members. The illness can also be dangerous. Some young people with bipolar disorder try to hurt themselves or attempt suicide.

About This Chapter: This chapter includes text excerpted from "Bipolar Disorder In Children And Teens," National Institute of Mental Health (NIMH), 2015.

Children and teens with bipolar disorder should get treatment. With help, they can manage their symptoms and lead successful lives.

Types Of Bipolar Disorder

There are four basic types of bipolar disorder; all of them involve clear changes in mood, energy, and activity levels. These moods range from periods of extremely "up," elated, and energized behavior (known as manic episodes) to very sad, "down," or hopeless periods (known as depressive episodes). Less severe manic periods are known as hypomanic episodes.

- **Bipolar I Disorder**—defined by manic episodes that last at least 7 days, or by manic symptoms that are so severe that the person needs immediate hospital care. Usually, depressive episodes occur as well, typically lasting at least 2 weeks. Episodes of depression with mixed features (having depression and manic symptoms at the same time) are also possible.

- **Bipolar II Disorder**—defined by a pattern of depressive episodes and hypomanic episodes, but not the full-blown manic episodes described above.

- **Cyclothymic Disorder (also called cyclothymia)**—defined by numerous periods of hypomanic symptoms as well numerous periods of depressive symptoms lasting for at least 2 years (1 year in children and adolescents). However, the symptoms do not meet the diagnostic requirements for a hypomanic episode and a depressive episode.

- **Other Specified and Unspecified Bipolar and Related Disorders**—defined by bipolar disorder symptoms that do not match the three categories listed above.

(Source: "Bipolar Disorder," National Institute of Mental Health (NIMH).)

Who Develops Bipolar Disorder?

Anyone can develop bipolar disorder, including children and teens. However, most people with bipolar disorder develop it in their late teen or early adult years. The illness usually lasts a lifetime.

Why Does Someone Develop Bipolar Disorder?

Doctors do not know what causes bipolar disorder, but several things may contribute to the illness. Family genes may be one factor because bipolar disorder sometimes runs in families. However, it is important to know that just because someone in your family has bipolar disorder, it does not mean other members of the family will have it as well.

Another factor that may lead to bipolar disorder is the brain structure or the brain function of the person with the disorder. Scientists are finding out more about the disorder by studying it. This research may help doctors do a better job of treating people. Also, this research may help doctors to predict whether a person will get bipolar disorder. One day, doctors may be able to prevent the illness in some people.

What Are The Symptoms Of Bipolar Disorder?

Bipolar "mood episodes" include unusual mood changes along with unusual sleep habits, activity levels, thoughts, or behavior. In a child, these mood and activity changes must be very different from their usual behavior and from the behavior of other children. A person with bipolar disorder may have manic episodes, depressive episodes, or "mixed" episodes. A mixed episode has both manic and depressive symptoms. These mood episodes cause symptoms that last a week or two or sometimes longer. During an episode, the symptoms last every day for most of the day.

Children and teens having a manic episode may:

- Feel very happy or act silly in a way that's unusual for them and for other people their age

- Have a very short temper

- Talk really fast about a lot of different things

- Have trouble sleeping but not feel tired

- Have trouble staying focused

- Talk and think about sex more often

- Do risky things

Children and teens having a depressive episode may:

- Feel very sad

- Complain about pain a lot, such as stomachaches and headaches

- Sleep too little or too much

- Feel guilty and worthless

- Eat too little or too much

- Have little energy and no interest in fun activities

- Think about death or suicide

Can Children And Teens With Bipolar Disorder Have Other Problems?

Young people with bipolar disorder can have several problems at the same time. These include:

- **Substance abuse.** Both adults and kids with bipolar disorder are at risk of drinking or taking drugs.

- **Attention deficit hyperactivity disorder (ADHD).** Children who have both bipolar disorder and ADHD may have trouble staying focused.

- **Anxiety disorders,** like separation anxiety.

Sometimes behavior problems go along with mood episodes. Young people may take a lot of risks, such as driving too fast or spending too much money. Some young people with bipolar disorder think about suicide. Watch for any signs of suicidal thinking. Take these signs seriously and call your child's doctor.

How Is Bipolar Disorder Diagnosed?

An experienced doctor will carefully examine your child. There are no blood tests or brain scans that can diagnose bipolar disorder. Instead, the doctor will ask questions about your child's mood and sleeping patterns. The doctor will also ask about your child's energy and behavior. Sometimes doctors need to know about medical problems in your family, such as depression or alcoholism. The doctor may use tests to see if something other than bipolar disorder is causing your child's symptoms.

How Is Bipolar Disorder Treated?

Right now, there is no cure for bipolar disorder. Doctors often treat children who have the illness in much the same way they treat adults. Treatment can help control symptoms. Steady, dependable treatment works better than treatment that starts and stops. Treatment options include:

- **Medication.** There are several types of medication that can help. Children respond to medications in different ways, so the right type of medication depends on the child. Some children may need more than one type of medication because their symptoms are so complex. Sometimes they need to try different types of medicine to see which are best for them. Children should take the fewest number of medications and the smallest doses possible to help their symptoms. A good way to remember this is "start low, go slow." Medications can cause side effects. Always tell your child's doctor about any problems with side effects. Do not stop giving your child medication without a doctor's help. Stopping medication suddenly can be dangerous, and it can make bipolar symptoms worse.

- **Therapy.** Different kinds of psychotherapy, or "talk" therapy, can help children with bipolar disorder. Therapy can help children change their behavior and manage their routines. It can also help young people get along better with family and friends. Sometimes therapy includes family members

What Can Children And Teens Expect From Treatment?

With treatment, children and teens with bipolar disorder can get better over time. It helps when doctors, parents, and young people work together.

Sometimes a child's bipolar disorder changes. When this happens, treatment needs to change too. For example, your child may need to try a different medication. The doctor may also recommend other treatment changes. Symptoms may come back after a while, and more adjustments may be needed. Treatment can take time, but sticking with it helps many children and teens have fewer bipolar symptoms.

You can help treatment be more effective. Try keeping a chart of your child's moods, behaviors, and sleep patterns. This is called a "daily life chart" or "mood chart." It can help you and your child understand and track the illness. A chart can also help the doctor see whether treatment is working.

How Can I Help My Child Or Teen?

Help begins with the right diagnosis and treatment. If you think your child may have bipolar disorder, make an appointment with your family doctor to talk about the symptoms you notice.

If your child has bipolar disorder, here are some basic things you can do:

- Be patient.

- Encourage your child to talk, and listen to your child carefully.

- Be understanding about mood episodes.

- Help your child have fun.

- Help your child understand that treatment can make life better.

How Does Bipolar Disorder Affect Parents And Family?

Taking care of a child or teenager with bipolar disorder can be stressful for you, too. You have to cope with the mood swings and other problems, such as short tempers and risky activities. This can challenge any parent. Sometimes the stress can strain your relationships with other people, and you may miss work or lose free time.

If you are taking care of a child with bipolar disorder, take care of yourself too. Find someone you can talk to about your feelings. Talk with the doctor about support groups for caregivers. If you keep your stress level down, you will do a better job. It might help your child get better too.

Where Do I Go For Help?

If you're not sure where to get help, call your family doctor. You can also check the phone book for mental health professionals. Hospital doctors can help in an emergency. Finally, the Substance Abuse and Mental Health Services Administration (SAMHSA) has an online tool to help you find mental health services in your area.

I Know Someone Who Is In Crisis. What Do I Do?

If you know someone who might be thinking about hurting himself or herself or someone else, get help quickly.

- Do not leave the person alone.

- Call your doctor.

- Call 911 or go to the emergency room.

- Call National Suicide Prevention Lifeline, toll-free: 1-800-273-TALK (1-800-273-8255).

Chapter 13

Generalized Anxiety Disorder: When Worry Gets Out Of Control

What Is Generalized Anxiety Disorder (GAD)?

Occasional anxiety is a normal part of life. You might worry about things like health, money, or family problems. But people with generalized anxiety disorder (GAD) feel extremely worried or feel nervous about these and other things—even when there is little or no reason to worry about them. People with GAD find it difficult to control their anxiety and stay focused on daily tasks.

People with generalized anxiety disorder (GAD) go through the day filled with exaggerated worry and tension, even though there is little or nothing to provoke it. They anticipate disaster and are overly concerned about health issues, money, family problems, or difficulties at work. Sometimes just the thought of getting through the day produces anxiety.

GAD is diagnosed when a person worries excessively about a variety of everyday problems for at least 6 months.13 People with GAD can't seem to get rid of their concerns, even though they usually realize that their anxiety is more intense than the situation warrants. They can't relax, startle easily, and have difficulty concentrating. Often they have trouble falling asleep or staying asleep. Physical symptoms that often accompany the anxiety include fatigue, headaches, muscle tension, muscle aches, difficulty swallowing, trembling, twitching, irritability, sweating, nausea, lightheadedness, having to go to the bathroom frequently, feeling out of breath, and hot flashes.

When their anxiety level is mild, people with GAD can function socially and hold down a job. Although they don't avoid certain situations as a result of their disorder, people with GAD can have difficulty carrying out the simplest daily activities if their anxiety is severe.

About This Chapter: This chapter includes text excerpted from "Generalized Anxiety Disorder: When Worry Gets Out Of Control," National Institute of Mental Health (NIMH), 2016.

GAD affects about 6.8 million American adults, including twice as many women as men. The disorder develops gradually and can begin at any point in the life cycle, although the years of highest risk are between childhood and middle age. There is evidence that genes play a modest role in GAD.

Other anxiety disorders, depression, or substance abuse often accompany GAD, which rarely occurs alone. GAD is commonly treated with medication or cognitive-behavioral therapy, but co-occurring conditions must also be treated using the appropriate therapies.

(Source: "Generalized Anxiety Disorder (GAD)," National Institute of Mental Health (NIMH).)

What Are The Signs And Symptoms Of GAD?

GAD develops slowly. It often starts during the teen years or young adulthood. People with GAD may:

- Worry very much about everyday things

- Have trouble controlling their worries or feelings of nervousness

- Know that they worry much more than they should

- Feel restless and have trouble relaxing

- Have a hard time concentrating

- Be easily startled

- Have trouble falling asleep or staying asleep

- Feel easily tired or tired all the time

- Have headaches, muscle aches, stomach aches, or unexplained pains

- Have a hard time swallowing

- Tremble or twitch

- Be irritable or feel "on edge"

- Sweat a lot, feel light-headed or out of breath

- Have to go to the bathroom a lot

Children and teens with GAD often worry excessively about:

- Their performance, such as in school or in sports

- Catastrophes, such as earthquakes or war

Both children and adults with GAD may experience physical symptoms that make it hard to function and that interfere with daily life.

> Symptoms may get better or worse at different times, and they are often worse during times of stress, such as with a physical illness, during exams at school, or during a family or relationship conflict.

What Causes GAD?

GAD sometimes runs in families, but no one knows for sure why some family members have it while others don't. Researchers have found that several parts of the brain, as well as biological processes, play a key role in fear and anxiety.

How Is GAD Treated?

First, talk to your doctor about your symptoms. Your doctor should do an exam and ask you about your health history to make sure that an unrelated physical problem is not causing your symptoms. Your doctor may refer to you a mental health specialist, such as a psychiatrist or psychologist.

GAD is generally treated with psychotherapy, medication, or both. Talk with your doctor about the best treatment for you.

Psychotherapy

A type of psychotherapy called cognitive behavioral therapy (CBT) is especially useful for treating GAD. CBT teaches a person different ways of thinking, behaving, and reacting to situations that help him or her feel less anxious and worried.

What Is It Like To Have GAD?

"I was worried all the time and felt nervous. My family told me that there were no signs of problems, but I still felt upset. I dreaded going to work because I couldn't keep my mind focused. I was having trouble falling asleep at night and was irritated at my family all the time.

I saw my doctor and explained my constant worries. My doctor sent me to someone who knows about GAD. Now I am working with a counselor to cope better with my anxiety. I had to work hard, but I feel better. I'm glad I made that first call to my doctor."

Medication

Doctors may also prescribe medication to help treat GAD. Your doctor will work with you to find the best medication and dose for you. Different types of medication can be effective in GAD:

- Selective serotonin reuptake inhibitors (SSRIs)

- Serotonin-norepinephrine reuptake inhibitors (SNRIs)

- Other serotonergic medication

- Benzodiazepines

Doctors commonly use SSRIs and SNRIs to treat depression, but they are also helpful for the symptoms of GAD. They may take several weeks to start working. These medications may also cause side effects, such as headaches, nausea, or difficulty sleeping. These side effects are usually not severe for most people, especially if the dose starts off low and is increased slowly over time.

Buspirone is another serotonergic medication that can be helpful in GAD. Buspirone needs to be taken continuously for several weeks for it to be fully effective.

Benzodiazepines, which are sedative medications, can also be used to manage severe forms of GAD. These medications are powerfully effective in rapidly decreasing anxiety, but they can cause tolerance and dependence if you use them continuously. Therefore, your doctor will only prescribe them for brief periods of time if you need them.

Chapter 14

Social Anxiety Disorder: Always Embarrassed

Are you extremely afraid of being judged by others?

Are you very self-conscious in everyday social situations?

Do you avoid meeting new people?

If you have been feeling this way for at least six months and these feelings make it hard for you to do everyday tasks—such as talking to people at work or school—you may have a social anxiety disorder.

Social anxiety disorder (also called social phobia) is a mental health condition. It is an intense, persistent fear of being watched and judged by others. This fear can affect work, school, and your other day-to-day activities. It can even make it hard to make and keep friends. But social anxiety disorder doesn't have to stop you from reaching your potential. Treatment can help you overcome your symptoms.

> Social phobia, also called social anxiety disorder, is diagnosed when people become overwhelmingly anxious and very self-conscious in everyday social situations. People with social phobia have a strong fear of being watched and judged by others and of doing things that will embarrass them. They can worry for days or weeks before a dreaded situation. This fear may become so severe that it interferes with work, school, and other ordinary activities, and can make it hard to make and keep friends.
>
> Social phobia affects about 15 million American adults and affects women and men in equal numbers. People with social phobia often have other anxiety disorders and/or depression as

About This Chapter: This chapter includes text excerpted from "Social Anxiety Disorder: More Than Just Shyness," National Institute of Mental Health (NIMH), November 2016.

well. Substance abuse can develop if a person with social phobia uses alcohol or drugs to soothe their anxiety.

(Source: "Mental Health," National Women's Health Information Center (NWHIC), Office on Women's Health (OWH).)

What Is Social Anxiety Disorder?

Social anxiety disorder is a common type of anxiety disorder. A person with social anxiety disorder feels symptoms of anxiety or fear in certain or all social situations, such as meeting new people, dating, being on a job interview, answering a question in class, or having to talk to a cashier in a store. Doing everyday things in front of people—such as eating or drinking in front of others or using a public restroom—also causes anxiety or fear. The person is afraid that he or she will be humiliated, judged, and rejected.

The fear that people with social anxiety disorder have in social situations is so strong that they feel it is beyond their ability to control. As a result, it gets in the way of going to work, attending school, or doing everyday things. People with social anxiety disorder may worry about these and other things for weeks before they happen. Sometimes, they end up staying away from places or events where they think they might have to do something that will embarrass them.

Some people with the disorder do not have anxiety in social situations but have performance anxiety instead. They feel physical symptoms of anxiety in situations such as giving a speech, playing a sports game, or dancing or playing a musical instrument on stage.

Social anxiety disorder usually starts during youth in people who are extremely shy. Social anxiety disorder is not uncommon; research suggests that about 7 percent of Americans are affected. Without treatment, social anxiety disorder can last for many years or a lifetime and prevent a person from reaching his or her full potential.

What Are The Signs And Symptoms Of Social Anxiety Disorder?

When having to perform in front of or be around others, people with social anxiety disorder tend to:

- Blush, sweat, tremble, feel a rapid heart rate, or feel their "mind going blank"

- Feel nauseous or sick to their stomach

- Show a rigid body posture, make little eye contact, or speak with an overly soft voice

- Find it scary and difficult to be with other people, especially those they don't already know, and have a hard time talking to them even though they wish they could

- Be very self-conscious in front of other people and feel embarrassed and awkward

- Be very afraid that other people will judge them

- Stay away from places where there are other people

What Causes Social Anxiety Disorder?

Social anxiety disorder sometimes runs in families, but no one knows for sure why some family members have it while others don't. Researchers have found that several parts of the brain are involved in fear and anxiety. Some researchers think that misreading of others' behavior may play a role in causing or worsening social anxiety. For example, you may think that people are staring or frowning at you when they truly are not. Underdeveloped social skills are another possible contributor to social anxiety. For example, if you have underdeveloped social skills, you may feel discouraged after talking with people and may worry about doing it in the future.

How Is Social Anxiety Disorder Treated?

First, talk to your doctor or healthcare professional about your symptoms. Your doctor should do an exam and ask you about your health history to make sure that an unrelated physical problem is not causing your symptoms. Your doctor may refer you to a mental health specialist, such as a psychiatrist, psychologist, clinical social worker, or counselor. The first step to effective treatment is to have a diagnosis made, usually by a mental health specialist.

Social anxiety disorder is generally treated with psychotherapy (sometimes called "talk" therapy), medication, or both. Speak with your doctor or healthcare provider about the best treatment for you.

Psychotherapy

A type of psychotherapy called cognitive behavioral therapy (CBT) is especially useful for treating social anxiety disorder. CBT teaches you different ways of thinking, behaving, and reacting to situations that help you feel less anxious and fearful. It can also help you learn and practice social skills. CBT delivered in a group format can be especially helpful.

What Is It Like Having Social Anxiety Disorder?

"In school, I was always afraid of being called on, even when I knew the answers. I didn't want people to think I was stupid or boring. My heart would pound and I would feel dizzy and sick. When I got a job, I hated to meet with my boss or talk in a meeting. I couldn't attend my best friend's wedding reception because I was afraid of having to meet new people. I tried to calm myself by drinking several glasses of wine before an event and then I started drinking every day to try to face what I had to do."

"I finally talked to my doctor because I was tired of feeling this way and I was worried that I would lose my job. I now take medicine and meet with a counselor to talk about ways to cope with my fears. I refuse to use alcohol to escape my fears and I'm on my way to feeling better."

Support Groups

Many people with social anxiety also find support groups helpful. In a group of people who all have social anxiety disorder, you can receive unbiased, honest feedback about how others in the group see you. This way, you can learn that your thoughts about judgment and rejection are not true or are distorted. You can also learn how others with social anxiety disorder approach and overcome the fear of social situations.

Medication

There are three types of medications used to help treat social anxiety disorder:

- Antianxiety medications

- Antidepressants

- Beta blockers

Antianxiety medications are powerful and begin working right away to reduce anxious feelings; however, these medications are usually not taken for long periods of time. People can buildup a tolerance if they are taken over a long period of time and may need higher and higher doses to get the same effect. Some people may even become dependent on them. To avoid these problems, doctors usually prescribe antianxiety medications for short periods, a practice that is especially helpful for older adults.

Antidepressants are mainly used to treat depression, but are also helpful for the symptoms of social anxiety disorder. In contrast to antianxiety medications, they may take several weeks to start working. Antidepressants may also cause side effects, such as headaches, nausea, or difficulty sleeping. These side effects are usually not severe for most people, especially if the dose starts off low and is increased slowly over time. Talk to your doctor about any side effects that you have.

Beta blockers are medicines that can help block some of the physical symptoms of anxiety on the body, such as an increased heart rate, sweating, or tremors. Beta blockers are commonly the medications of choice for the "performance anxiety" type of social anxiety.

Your doctor will work with you to find the best medication, dose, and duration of treatment. Many people with social anxiety disorder obtain the best results with a combination of medication and CBT or other psychotherapies.

Don't give up on treatment too quickly. Both psychotherapy and medication can take some time to work. A healthy lifestyle can also help combat anxiety. Make sure to get enough sleep and exercise, eat a healthy diet, and turn to family and friends who you trust for support.

Chapter 15

Posttraumatic Stress Disorder

Posttraumatic stress disorder (PTSD) is a disorder that develops in some people who have experienced a shocking, scary, or dangerous event.

It is natural to feel afraid during and after a traumatic situation. Fear triggers many split-second changes in the body to help defend against danger or to avoid it. This "fight-or-flight" response is a typical reaction meant to protect a person from harm. Nearly everyone will experience a range of reactions after trauma, yet most people recover from initial symptoms naturally. Those who continue to experience problems may be diagnosed with PTSD. People who have PTSD may feel stressed or frightened even when they are not in danger.

Signs And Symptoms Of Posttraumatic Stress Disorder (PTSD)

Not every traumatized person develops ongoing (chronic) or even short-term (acute) PTSD. Not everyone with PTSD has been through a dangerous event. Some experiences, like the sudden, unexpected death of a loved one, can also cause PTSD. Symptoms usually begin early, within 3 months of the traumatic incident, but sometimes they begin years afterward. Symptoms must last more than a month and be severe enough to interfere with relationships or work to be considered PTSD. The course of the illness varies. Some people recover within 6 months, while others have symptoms that last much longer. In some people, the condition becomes chronic.

About This Chapter: This chapter includes text excerpted from "Post-Traumatic Stress Disorder," National Institute of Mental Health (NIMH), February 2016.

A doctor who has experience helping people with mental illnesses, such as a psychiatrist or psychologist, can diagnose PTSD.

To be diagnosed with PTSD, an adult must have all of the following for at least 1 month:

- At least one re-experiencing symptom
- At least one avoidance symptom
- At least two arousal and reactivity symptoms
- At least two cognition and mood symptoms

Re-experiencing symptoms include:

- Flashbacks—reliving the trauma over and over, including physical symptoms like a racing heart or sweating
- Bad dreams
- Frightening thoughts

Re-experiencing symptoms may cause problems in a person's everyday routine. The symptoms can start from the person's own thoughts and feelings. Words, objects, or situations that are reminders of the event can also trigger re-experiencing symptoms.

Avoidance symptoms include:

- Staying away from places, events, or objects that are reminders of the traumatic experience
- Avoiding thoughts or feelings related to the traumatic event

Things that remind a person of the traumatic event can trigger avoidance symptoms. These symptoms may cause a person to change his or her personal routine. For example, after a bad car accident, a person who usually drives may avoid driving or riding in a car.

Arousal and reactivity symptoms include:

- Being easily startled
- Feeling tense or "on edge"
- Having difficulty sleeping
- Having angry outbursts

Arousal symptoms are usually constant, instead of being triggered by things that remind one of the traumatic events. These symptoms can make the person feel stressed and angry. They may make it hard to do daily tasks, such as sleeping, eating, or concentrating.

Cognition and mood symptoms include:

- Trouble remembering key features of the traumatic event

- Negative thoughts about oneself or the world

- Distorted feelings like guilt or blame

- Loss of interest in enjoyable activities

Cognition and mood symptoms can begin or worsen after the traumatic event, but are not due to injury or substance use. These symptoms can make the person feel alienated or detached from friends or family members.

It is natural to have some of these symptoms after a dangerous event. Sometimes people have very serious symptoms that go away after a few weeks. This is called acute stress disorder, or ASD. When the symptoms last more than a month, seriously affect one's ability to function, and are not due to substance use, medical illness, or anything except the event itself, they might be PTSD. Some people with PTSD don't show any symptoms for weeks or months. PTSD is often accompanied by depression, substance abuse, or one or more of the other anxiety disorders.

Do Children React Differently Than Adults?

Children and teens can have extreme reactions to trauma, but their symptoms may not be the same as adults. In very young children (less than 6 years of age), these symptoms can include:

- Wetting the bed after having learned to use the toilet

- Forgetting how to or being unable to talk

- Acting out the scary event during playtime

- Being unusually clingy with a parent or other adult

Older children and teens are more likely to show symptoms similar to those seen in adults. They may also develop disruptive, disrespectful, or destructive behaviors. Older children and teens may feel guilty for not preventing injury or deaths. They may also have thoughts of revenge.

Risk Factors Of PTSD

Anyone can develop PTSD at any age. This includes war veterans, children, and people who have been through a physical or sexual assault, abuse, accident, disaster, or many other serious events. According to the National Center for PTSD, about 7 or 8 out of every 100 people will experience PTSD at some point in their lives. Women are more likely to develop PTSD than men, and genes may make some people more likely to develop PTSD than others.

Not everyone with PTSD has been through a dangerous event. Some people develop PTSD after a friend or family member experiences danger or harm. The sudden, unexpected death of a loved one can also lead to PTSD.

Why Do Some People Develop PTSD And Other People Do Not?

It is important to remember that not everyone who lives through a dangerous event develops PTSD. In fact, most people will not develop the disorder.

Many factors play a part in whether a person will develop PTSD. Some examples are listed below. Risk factors make a person more likely to develop PTSD. Other factors, called resilience factors, can help reduce the risk of the disorder.

Risk Factors And Resilience Factors For PTSD

Some factors that increase risk for PTSD include:

- Living through dangerous events and traumas

- Getting hurt

- Seeing another person hurt, or seeing a dead body

- Childhood trauma

- Feeling horror, helplessness, or extreme fear

- Having little or no social support after the event

- Dealing with extra stress after the event, such as loss of a loved one, pain and injury, or loss of a job or home

- Having a history of mental illness or substance abuse

Some resilience factors that may reduce the risk of PTSD include:

- Seeking out support from other people, such as friends and family

- Finding a support group after a traumatic event

- Learning to feel good about one's own actions in the face of danger

- Having a positive coping strategy, or a way of getting through the bad event and learning from it

- Being able to act and respond effectively despite feeling fear

Researchers are studying the importance of these and other risk and resilience factors, including genetics and neurobiology. With more research, someday it may be possible to predict who is likely to develop PTSD and to prevent it.

How Is PTSD Measured?

- To develop PTSD, a person must have gone through a trauma. Almost all people who go through trauma have some symptoms for a short time after the trauma. Yet most people do not get PTSD. A certain pattern of symptoms is involved in PTSD. There are four major types of symptoms: re-experiencing, avoidance, arousal, and negative changes in beliefs and feelings.

- Deciding if someone has PTSD can involve several steps. The diagnosis of PTSD is most often made by a mental health provider. To diagnose PTSD, a mental health provider "measures," "assesses," or "evaluates" PTSD symptoms you may have had since the trauma.

(Source: "How Is PTSD Measured?" National Center for Posttraumatic Stress Disorder (NCPTSD), U.S. Department of Veterans Affairs (VA).)

Treatments And Therapies Of PTSD

The main treatments for people with PTSD are medications, psychotherapy ("talk" therapy), or both. Everyone is different, and PTSD affects people differently so a treatment that works for one person may not work for another. It is important for anyone with PTSD to be treated by a mental health provider who is experienced with PTSD. Some people with PTSD need to try different treatments to find what works for their symptoms.

If someone with PTSD is going through an ongoing trauma, such as being in an abusive relationship, both of the problems need to be addressed. Other ongoing problems can include panic disorder, depression, substance abuse, and feeling suicidal.

Medications

The most studied medications for treating PTSD include antidepressants, which may help control PTSD symptoms such as sadness, worry, anger, and feeling numb inside. Antidepressants and other medications may be prescribed along with psychotherapy.

Psychotherapy

Psychotherapy (sometimes called "talk therapy") involves talking with a mental health professional to treat a mental illness. Psychotherapy can occur one-on-one or in a group. Talk therapy treatment for PTSD usually lasts 6 to 12 weeks, but it can last longer. Research shows that support from family and friends can be an important part of recovery.

Many types of psychotherapy can help people with PTSD. Some types target the symptoms of PTSD directly. Other therapies focus on social, family, or job-related problems. The doctor or therapist may combine different therapies depending on each person's needs.

Effective psychotherapies tend to emphasize a few key components, including education about symptoms, teaching skills to help identify the triggers of symptoms, and skills to manage the symptoms. One helpful form of therapy is called cognitive behavioral therapy, or CBT. CBT can include:

- **Exposure therapy.** This helps people face and control their fear. It gradually exposes them to the trauma they experienced in a safe way. It uses imagining, writing, or visiting the place where the event happened. The therapist uses these tools to help people with PTSD cope with their feelings.

- **Cognitive restructuring.** This helps people make sense of the bad memories. Sometimes people remember the event differently than how it happened. They may feel guilt or shame about something that is not their fault. The therapist helps people with PTSD look at what happened in a realistic way.

There are other types of treatment that can help as well. People with PTSD should talk about all treatment options with a therapist. Treatment should equip individuals with the skills to manage their symptoms and help them participate in activities that they enjoyed before developing PTSD.

How Talk Therapies Help People Overcome PTSD

Talk therapies teach people helpful ways to react to the frightening events that trigger their PTSD symptoms. Based on this general goal, different types of therapy may:

- Teach about trauma and its effects

- Use relaxation and anger-control skills

- Provide tips for better sleep, diet, and exercise habits

- Help people identify and deal with guilt, shame, and other feelings about the event

- Focus on changing how people react to their PTSD symptoms. For example, therapy helps people face reminders of the trauma.

Beyond Treatment: How Can I Help Myself?

It may be very hard to take that first step to help yourself. It is important to realize that although it may take some time, with treatment, you can get better. If you are unsure where to go for help, ask your family doctor. You can also check National Institute of Mental Health's (NIMH) Help for Mental Illnesses page or search online for "mental health providers," "social services," "hotlines," or "physicians" for phone numbers and addresses. An emergency room doctor can also provide temporary help and can tell you where and how to get further help.

To help yourself while in treatment:

- Talk with your doctor about treatment options

- Engage in mild physical activity or exercise to help reduce stress

- Set realistic goals for yourself

- Break up large tasks into small ones, set some priorities, and do what you can as you can

- Try to spend time with other people, and confide in a trusted friend or relative. Tell others about things that may trigger symptoms.

- Expect your symptoms to improve gradually, not immediately

- Identify and seek out comforting situations, places, and people

Caring for yourself and others is especially important when large numbers of people are exposed to traumatic events (such as natural disasters, accidents, and violent acts).

Chapter 16

Obsessive-Compulsive Disorder: When Unwanted Thoughts Take Over

Do you constantly have disturbing uncontrollable thoughts? Do you feel the urge to repeat the same behaviors or rituals over and over? Are these thoughts and behaviors making it hard for you to do things you enjoy?

If so, you may have obsessive-compulsive disorder (OCD). The good news is that, with treatment, you can overcome the fears and behaviors that may be putting your life on hold.

What Is It Like To Have Obsessive-Compulsive Disorder (OCD)?

"I couldn't do anything without my rituals. They invaded every aspect of my life. Counting really bogged me down. I would wash my hair three times because three was a good luck number for me. It took me longer to read because I'd have to count the lines in a paragraph. When I set my alarm at night, I had to set it to a time that wouldn't add up to a 'bad' number."

"Getting dressed in the morning was tough because I had to follow my routine or I would become very anxious and start getting dressed all over again." I always worried that if I didn't follow my routine, my parents were going to die. These thoughts triggered more anxiety and more rituals. Because of the time I spent on rituals, I was unable to do a lot of things that were important to me. I couldn't seem to overcome them until I got treatment."

About This Chapter: This chapter includes text excerpted from "Obsessive-Compulsive Disorder: When Unwanted Thoughts Or Irresistible Actions Take Over," National Institute of Mental Health (NIMH), 2016.

What Is Obsessive-Compulsive Disorder (OCD)?

OCD is a common, chronic (long-lasting) disorder in which a person has uncontrollable, reoccurring thoughts (obsessions) and behaviors (compulsions) that he or she feels the urge to repeat over and over in response to the obsession.

While everyone sometimes feels the need to double check things, people with OCD have uncontrollable thoughts that cause them anxiety, urging them to check things repeatedly or perform routines and rituals for at least 1 hour per day. Performing the routines or rituals may bring brief but temporary relief from the anxiety. However, left untreated, these thoughts and rituals cause the person great distress and get in the way of work, school, and personal relationships.

What Are The Signs And Symptoms Of OCD?

People with OCD may have obsessions, compulsions, or both. Some people with OCD also have a tic disorder. Motor tics are sudden, brief, repetitive movements, such as eye blinking, facial grimacing, shoulder shrugging, or head or shoulder jerking. Common vocal tics include repetitive throat-clearing, sniffing, or grunting sounds.

Obsessions may include:

- Fear of germs or contamination

- Fear of losing or misplacing something

- Worries about harm coming towards oneself or others

- Unwanted and taboo thoughts involving sex, religion, or others

- Having things symmetrical or in perfect order

Compulsions may include:

- Excessively cleaning or washing a body part

- Keeping or hoarding unnecessary objects

- Ordering or arranging items in a particular, precise way

- Repeatedly checking on things, such as making sure that the door is locked or the oven is off

- Repeatedly counting items

- Constantly seeking reassurance

What Causes OCD?

OCD may have a genetic component. It sometimes runs in families, but no one knows for sure why some family members have it while others don't. OCD usually begins in adolescence or young adulthood, and tends to appear at a younger age in boys than in girls. Researchers have found that several parts of the brain, as well as biological processes, play a key role in obsessive thoughts and compulsive behavior, as well as the fear and anxiety related to them. Researchers also know that people who have suffered physical or sexual trauma are at an increased risk for OCD.

Some children may develop a sudden onset or worsening of OCD symptoms after a streptococcal infection; this postinfectious autoimmune syndrome is called Pediatric Autoimmune Neuropsychiatric Disorder Associated with Streptococcal Infections (PANDAS).

How Is OCD Treated?

The first step is to talk with your doctor or healthcare provider about your symptoms. The clinician should do an exam and ask you about your health history to make sure that a physical problem is not causing your symptoms. Your doctor may refer you to a mental health specialist, such as a psychiatrist, psychologist, social worker, or counselor for further evaluation or treatment.

OCD is generally treated with cognitive behavior therapy, medication, or both. Speak with your mental health professional about the best treatment for you.

Cognitive Behavioral Therapy (CBT)

In general, CBT teaches you different ways of thinking, behaving, and reacting to the obsessions and compulsions.

Exposure and Response Prevention (EX/RP) is a specific form of CBT which has been shown to help many patients recover from OCD. EX/RP involves gradually exposing you to your fears or obsessions and teaching you healthy ways to deal with the anxiety they cause.

Other therapies, such as habit reversal training, can also help you overcome compulsions.

For children, mental health professionals can also identify strategies to manage stress and increase support to avoid exacerbating OCD symptoms in school and home settings.

Medication

Doctors also may prescribe different types of medications to help treat OCD including selective serotonin reuptake inhibitors (SSRIs) and a type of serotonin reuptake inhibitor (SRI) called clomipramine.

SSRIs and SRIs are commonly used to treat depression, but they are also helpful for the symptoms of OCD. SSRIs and SRIs may take 10–12 weeks to start working, longer than is required for the treatment of depression. These medications may also cause side effects, such as headaches, nausea, or difficulty sleeping.

People taking clomipramine, which is in a different class of medication from the SSRIs, sometimes experience dry mouth, constipation, rapid heartbeat, and dizziness on standing. These side effects are usually not severe for most people and improve as treatment continues, especially if the dose starts off low and is increased slowly over time. Talk to your doctor about any side effects that you have. Don't stop taking your medication without talking to your doctor first. Your doctor will work with you to find the best medication and dose for you.

Don't give up on treatment too quickly. Both psychotherapy and medication can take some time to work. While there is no cure for OCD, current treatments enable most people with this disorder to control their symptoms and lead full, productive lives. A healthy lifestyle that involves relaxation and managing stress can also help combat OCD. Make sure to also get enough sleep and exercise, eat a healthy diet, and turn to family and friends whom you trust for support.

Finding Help

Asking questions and providing information to your doctor or healthcare provider can improve your care. Talking with your doctor builds trust and leads to better results, quality, safety, and satisfaction.

Mental Health Treatment Program Locator

The Substance Abuse and Mental Health Services Administration (SAMHSA) provides this online resource for locating mental health treatment facilities and programs. The Mental Health Treatment Locator section of the Behavioral Health Treatment Services Locator lists facilities providing mental health services to persons with mental illness. Find a facility in your state at www.findtreatment.samhsa.gov.

Chapter 17

Phobias And Fears

Do you feel very afraid of, or feel a need to avoid, any of the objects or situations below? If you answered "yes" and have found that the fear or avoidance of one or more of these situations is getting in your way, you may consider speaking with your physician or mental health professional about your concerns.

- Animals (such as snakes, spiders, dogs, insects)
- Driving
- Heights, storms or water
- Enclosed places (such as elevators)
- Blood or needles
- Air travel
- Some other object or situation

(Source: "Specific Phobias," U.S. Department of Veterans Affairs (VA).)

A phobia is a type of anxiety disorder. It is a strong, irrational fear of something that poses little or no real danger. There are many specific phobias. Acrophobia is a fear of heights. Agoraphobia is a fear of public places, and claustrophobia is a fear of closed-in places. If you

About This Chapter: Text in this chapter begins with excerpts from "Phobias," National Institute of Mental Health (NIMH), August 9, 2016; Text under the heading "Specific Phobias" is excerpted from "Mental Health—Specific Phobias," Office on Women's Health (OWH), U.S. Department of Health and Human Services (HHS), March 29, 2010. Reviewed July 2017; Text under the heading "Specific Phobia Among Children" is excerpted from "Specific Phobia Among Children," National Institute of Mental Health (NIMH), July 18, 2014; Text under the heading "Nomophobia—A Potential New Phobia" is excerpted from "Are You Addicted To Your Cell Phone?" National Institute on Drug Abuse (NIDA) for Teens, February 14, 2013. Reviewed July 2017.

become anxious and extremely self-conscious in everyday social situations, you could have a social phobia. Other common phobias involve tunnels, highway driving, water, flying, animals, and blood.

People with phobias try to avoid what they are afraid of. If they cannot, they may experience:

- Panic and fear
- Rapid heartbeat
- Shortness of breath
- Trembling
- A strong desire to get away

Phobias usually start in children or teens, and continue into adulthood. The causes of specific phobias are not known, but they sometimes run in families. Treatment helps most people with phobias. Options include medicines, therapy or both.

Specific Phobias

A specific phobia is a strong, irrational fear of something that poses little or no actual danger. Some of the more common specific phobias are:

- Closed-in places
- Heights
- Escalators
- Tunnels
- Highway driving
- Water
- Flying
- Dogs
- Injuries involving blood

Such phobias aren't just extreme fear; they are irrational fear of a particular thing. You may be able to ski the world's tallest mountains with ease but be unable to go above the fifth floor of an office building. While adults with phobias realize that these fears are irrational, they often find that facing, or even thinking about facing, the feared object or situation brings on a panic attack or severe anxiety.

Specific phobias affect an estimated 19.2 million adult Americans and are twice as common in women as men. They usually appear in childhood or adolescence and tend to persist into adulthood. The causes of specific phobias are not well understood, but there is some evidence that the tendency to develop them may run in families.

If the feared situation or feared object is easy to avoid, people with specific phobias may not seek help. Treatment is needed if the phobia hurts a person's career or personal life.

Treatment

If you think you have an anxiety disorder such as specific phobia, the first person you should see is your family doctor. A physician can determine whether the symptoms that alarm you are due to an anxiety disorder, another medical condition, or both.

Specific phobias respond very well to carefully targeted psychotherapy.

Specific Phobia Among Teens

Specific phobia involves marked and persistent fear and avoidance of a specific object or situation. This type of phobia includes, but is not limited to, the fear of heights, spiders, and flying.

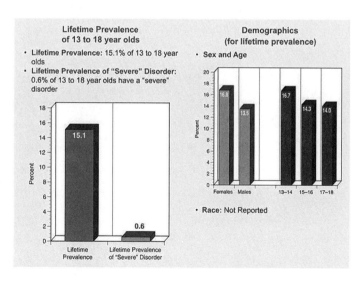

Figure 17.1. Specific Phobia

Nomophobia—A Potential New Phobia

Nomophobia—an abbreviation of "no-mobile-phone-phobia"—is also called "cell phone addiction." Symptoms include:

- Experiencing anxiety or panic over losing your phone

- Obsessively checking for missed calls, emails, and texts

- Using your phone in inappropriate places like the bathroom or church

- Missing out on opportunities for face-to-face interactions

A survey found that two-thirds of people in the United Kingdom experience nomophobia. That number increases to 77 percent for young people age 18–24. Cell phone use is definitely increasing everywhere, especially among teens—overall in the United States, 75 percent of all teens text, sending an average of 60–100 texts per day.

Researchers debate whether nomophobia is a real addiction. Addiction to drugs stems from their causing dopamine to flood the brain—which can trigger euphoria and a strong desire to repeat the experience. Researchers question whether the anticipation or rush of receiving an email, text, or Facebook status update may also trigger release of dopamine. But no studies have examined the issue.

Chapter 18

Panic Disorder: When Fear Overwhelms

Do you sometimes have sudden attacks of anxiety and overwhelming fear that last for several minutes? Maybe your heart pounds, you sweat, and you feel like you can't breathe or think. Do these attacks occur at unpredictable times with no obvious trigger, causing you to worry about the possibility of having another one at any time?

If so, you may have a type of anxiety disorder called panic disorder. Left untreated, panic disorder can lower your quality of life because it may lead to other fears and mental health disorders, problems at work or school, and social isolation.

What Is It Like To Have Panic Disorder?

"One day, without any warning or reason, a feeling of terrible anxiety came crashing down on me. I felt like I couldn't get enough air, no matter how hard I breathed. My heart was pounding out of my chest, and I thought I might die. I was sweating and felt dizzy. I felt like I had no control over these feelings and like I was drowning and couldn't think straight.

"After what seemed like an eternity, my breathing slowed and I eventually let go of the fear and my racing thoughts, but I was totally drained and exhausted. These attacks started to occur every couple of weeks, and I thought I was losing my mind. My friend saw how I was struggling and told me to call my doctor for help."

What Is Panic Disorder?

People with panic disorder have sudden and repeated attacks of fear that last for several minutes or longer. These are called panic attacks. Panic attacks are characterized by a fear of

---

About This Chapter: This chapter includes text excerpted from "Panic Disorder: When Fear Overwhelms," National Institute of Mental Health (NIMH), 2016.

disaster or of losing control even when there is no real danger. A person may also have a strong physical reaction during a panic attack. It may feel like having a heart attack. Panic attacks can occur at any time, and many people with panic disorder worry about and dread the possibility of having another attack.

A person with panic disorder may become discouraged and feel ashamed because he or she cannot carry out normal routines like going to school or work, going to the grocery store, or driving.

Panic disorder often begins in the late teens or early adulthood. More women than men have panic disorder. But not everyone who experiences panic attacks will develop panic disorder.

What Causes Panic Disorder?

Panic disorder sometimes runs in families, but no one knows for sure why some family members have it while others don't. Researchers have found that several parts of the brain, as well as biological processes, play a key role in fear and anxiety. Some researchers think that people with panic disorder misinterpret harmless bodily sensations as threats. By learning more about how the brain and body functions in people with panic disorder, scientists may be able to create better treatments. Researchers are also looking for ways in which stress and environmental factors may play a role.

What Are The Signs And Symptoms Of Panic Disorder?

People with panic disorder may have:

- Sudden and repeated panic attacks of overwhelming anxiety and fear

- A feeling of being out of control, or a fear of death or impending doom during a panic attack

- Physical symptoms during a panic attack, such as a pounding or racing heart, sweating, chills, trembling, breathing problems, weakness or dizziness, tingly or numb hands, chest pain, stomach pain, and nausea

- An intense worry about when the next panic attack will happen

- A fear or avoidance of places where panic attacks have occurred in the past

How Is Panic Disorder Treated?

First, talk to your doctor about your symptoms. Your doctor should do an exam and ask you about your health history to make sure that an unrelated physical problem is not causing your symptoms. Your doctor may refer to you a mental health specialist, such as a psychiatrist or psychologist.

Panic disorder is generally treated with psychotherapy, medication, or both. Talk with your doctor about the best treatment for you.

Psychotherapy. A type of psychotherapy called cognitive behavioral therapy (CBT) is especially useful as a first-line treatment for panic disorder. CBT teaches you different ways of thinking, behaving, and reacting to the feelings that come on with a panic attack. The attacks can begin to disappear once you learn to react differently to the physical sensations of anxiety and fear that occur during panic attacks.

Medication. Doctors also may prescribe different types of medications to help treat panic disorder:

- Selective serotonin reuptake inhibitors (SSRIs)

- Serotonin-norepinephrine reuptake inhibitors (SNRIs)

- Beta blockers

- Benzodiazepines

SSRIs and SNRIs are commonly used to treat depression, but they are also helpful for the symptoms of panic disorder. They may take several weeks to start working. These medications may also cause side-effects, such as headaches, nausea, or difficulty sleeping. These side effects are usually not severe for most people, especially if the dose starts off low and is increased slowly over time. Talk to your doctor about any side effects that you have.

Another type of medication called beta blockers can help control some of the physical symptoms of panic disorder, such as rapid heart rate. Although doctors do not commonly prescribe beta blockers for panic disorder, they may be helpful in certain situations that precede a panic attack.

Benzodiazepines, which are sedative medications, are powerfully effective in rapidly decreasing panic attack symptoms, but they can cause tolerance and dependence if you use them continuously. Therefore, your doctor will only prescribe them for brief periods of time if you need them.

Part Three
Personality And Psychotic Disorders

Chapter 19

Antisocial Personality Disorders

Antisocial personality disorder (ASPD) is a mental health condition in which a person has a long-term pattern of manipulating, exploiting, or violating the rights of others. This behavior is often criminal.

> Antisocial personality disorder is defined by the American Psychiatric Association's *Diagnostic and Statistical Manual of Mental Disorders, Fourth Edition* (DSM-IV) as "...a pervasive pattern of disregard for, and violation of, the rights of others that begins in childhood or early adolescence and continues into adulthood." People with antisocial personality disorder may disregard social norms and laws, repeatedly lie, place others at risk for their own benefit, and demonstrate a profound lack of remorse. It is sometimes referred to as sociopathic personality disorder, or sociopathy.
>
> *(Source: "Antisocial Personality Disorder," National Institute of Mental Health (NIMH).)*

Causes Of Antisocial Personality Disorders (ASPDs)

Cause of antisocial personality disorder is unknown. Genetic factors and environmental factors, such as child abuse, are believed to contribute to the development of this condition. People with an antisocial or alcoholic parent are at increased risk. Far more men than women are affected. The condition is common among people who are in prison.

Fire-setting and cruelty to animals during childhood are linked to the development of antisocial personality.

About This Chapter: Text in this chapter begins with excerpts from "Antisocial Personality Disorder," MentalHealth. gov, U.S. Department of Health and Human Services (HHS), January 4, 2013. Reviewed July 2017; Text under the heading "Treatment For ASPDs" is © 2017 Omnigraphics. Reviewed July 2017.

Some doctors believe that psychopathic personality (psychopathy) is the same disorder. Others believe that psychopathic personality is a similar but more severe disorder.

Symptoms Of ASPDs

A person with antisocial personality disorder may:

- Be able to act witty and charming

- Be good at flattery and manipulating other people's emotions

- Break the law repeatedly

- Disregard the safety of self and others

- Have problems with substance abuse

- Lie, steal, and fight often

- Not show guilt or remorse

- Often be angry or arrogant

12-month prevalence: 1 percent of U.S. adult population.

Demographics (for lifetime prevalence): There was a statistical trend for men to be more likely to have antisocial personality disorder than women.

12-month any service use (including healthcare): 46.1% of those with disorder are receiving treatment.

(Source: "Antisocial Personality Disorder," National Institute of Mental Health (NIMH).)

Treatment For ASPDs

Antisocial personality disorder is extremely difficult to treat, as there is no single solution. Also, any treatment requires long-term, close follow-up by experienced medical and mental health professionals. Individuals with this disorder rarely come forward for treatment and receive help, and even if they agree to treatment, they will attend therapy sessions irregularly and will likely drop out.

Most treatment programs focus on the following core issues:

- Modifying antisocial behavior

- Reducing criminal recidivism

- Any underlying, coexisting conditions such as substance abuse

Cognitive behavioral therapy (CBT) has been widely used and is found in some cases to be an effective one. CBT emphasizes behavior modification and teaches new coping mechanisms.

Psychotherapy, also called talk therapy, is sometimes used to treat antisocial personality disorder. Therapy will focus on anger and violence management, treatment for substance abuse, and other mental health conditions. This may not be as effective with severe symptoms of antisocial personality disorder.

Other complimentary methods as mindfulness techniques, yoga or meditation, hypnotism, and herbal remedies can helping some patients learn how to control emotions when faced with stressors.

No specific medications are approved for the treatment of antisocial personality disorder. Sometimes, medications are prescribed for the underlying coexisting mental health disorders such as anxiety, depression, or aggression.

References

1. "Antisocial Personality," GoodTherapy.org, July 3, 2015.

2. "Antisocial Personality Disorder," Mayo Clinic, April 2, 2016.

Chapter 20

Borderline Personality Disorder

Borderline personality disorder (BPD) is a serious mental disorder marked by a pattern of ongoing instability in moods, behavior, self-image, and functioning. These experiences often result in impulsive actions and unstable relationships. A person with BPD may experience intense episodes of anger, depression, and anxiety that may last from only a few hours to days.

Some people with BPD also have high rates of cooccurring mental disorders, such as mood disorders, anxiety disorders, and eating disorders, along with substance abuse, self-harm, suicidal thinking and behaviors, and suicide. While mental health experts now generally agree that the label "borderline personality disorder" is very misleading, a more accurate term does not exist yet.

Signs And Symptoms Of Borderline Personality Disorder (BPD)

People with BPD may experience extreme mood swings and can display uncertainty about who they are. As a result, their interests and values can change rapidly.

Other symptoms include:

- Frantic efforts to avoid real or imagined abandonment

- A pattern of intense and unstable relationships with family, friends, and loved ones, often swinging from extreme closeness and love (idealization) to extreme dislike or anger (devaluation)

- Distorted and unstable self-image or sense of self

About This Chapter: This chapter includes text excerpted from "Borderline Personality Disorder," National Institute of Mental Health (NIMH), August 2016.

- Impulsive and often dangerous behaviors, such as spending sprees, unsafe sex, substance abuse, reckless driving, and binge eating

- Recurring suicidal behaviors or threats or self-harming behavior, such as cutting

- Intense and highly changeable moods, with each episode lasting from a few hours to a few days

- Chronic feelings of emptiness

- Inappropriate, intense anger, or problems controlling anger

- Having stress-related paranoid thoughts

- Having severe dissociative symptoms, such as feeling cut off from oneself, observing oneself from outside the body, or losing touch with reality

Seemingly ordinary events may trigger symptoms. For example, people with BPD may feel angry and distressed over minor separations—such as vacations, business trips, or sudden changes of plans—from people to whom they feel close. Studies show that people with this disorder may see anger in an emotionally neutral face and have a stronger reaction to words with negative meanings than people who do not have the disorder.

Some of these signs and symptoms may be experienced by people with other mental health problems—and even by people without mental illness—and do not necessarily mean that they have BPD. It is important that a qualified and licensed mental health professional conduct a thorough assessment to determine whether or not a diagnosis of BPD or other mental disorder is warranted, and to help guide treatment options when appropriate.

Tests And Diagnosis Of BPD

Unfortunately, BPD is often underdiagnosed or misdiagnosed. A licensed mental health professional experienced in diagnosing and treating mental disorders—such as a psychiatrist, psychologist, or clinical social worker—can diagnose BPD based on a thorough interview and a comprehensive medical exam, which can help rule out other possible causes of symptoms.

The licensed mental health professional may ask about symptoms and personal and family medical histories, including any history of mental illnesses. This information can help the mental health professional decide on the best treatment. In some cases, cooccurring mental illnesses may have symptoms that overlap with BPD, making it difficult to distinguish BPD from other mental illnesses. For example, a person may describe feelings of depression but may not bring other symptoms to the mental health professional's attention.

Research funded by National Institute of Mental Health (NIMH) is underway to look for ways to improve diagnosis of and treatments for BPD, and to understand the various components of BPD and other personality disorders such as impulsivity, relationship problems, and emotional instability.

Risk Factors Of BPD

The causes of BPD are not yet clear, but research suggests that genetic, brain, environmental, and social factors are likely to be involved.

- **Genetics.** BPD is about five times more likely to occur if a person has a close family member (first-degree biological relatives) with the disorder.

- **Environmental and social factors.** Many people with BPD report experiencing traumatic life events, such as abuse or abandonment during childhood. Others may have been exposed to unstable relationships and hostile conflicts. However, some people with BPD do not have a history of trauma. And, many people with a history of traumatic life events do not have BPD.

- **Brain factors.** Studies show that people with BPD have structural and functional changes in the brain, especially in the areas that control impulses and emotional regulation. However, some people with similar changes in the brain do not have BPD. More research is needed to understand the relationship between brain structure and function and BPD.

Cause of borderline personality disorder is unknown. Genetic, family, and social factors are thought to play roles.

Risk factors for BPD include:

- Abandonment in childhood or adolescence
- Disrupted family life
- Poor communication in the family
- Sexual, physical, or emotional abuse

This personality disorder tends to occur more often in women and among hospitalized psychiatric patients.

(Source: "Borderline Personality Disorder," MentalHealth.gov, U.S. Department of Health and Human Services (HHS).)

Treatments And Therapies Of BPD

BPD has historically been viewed as difficult to treat. However, with newer and proper treatment, many people with BPD experience fewer or less severe symptoms and an improved quality of life. Many factors affect the length of time it takes for symptoms to improve once treatment begins, so it is important for people with BPD and their loved ones to be patient and to receive appropriate support during treatment. People with BPD can recover.

Psychotherapy

Psychotherapy (or "talk therapy") is the main treatment for people with BPD. Psychotherapy can be provided one-on-one between the therapist and the patient or in a group setting. Therapist-led group sessions may help teach people with BPD how to interact with others and how to express themselves effectively. It is important that people in therapy get along with and trust their therapist. The very nature of BPD can make it difficult for people with this disorder to maintain a comfortable and trusting bond with their therapist.

Types of psychotherapy used to treat BPD include:

- **Cognitive Behavioral Therapy (CBT):** Cognitive behavioral therapy (CBT) can help people with BPD identify and change core beliefs and/or behaviors that underlie inaccurate perceptions of themselves and others and problems interacting with others. CBT may help reduce a range of mood and anxiety symptoms and reduce the number of suicidal or self-harming behaviors.

- **Dialectical Behavior Therapy (DBT):** This type of therapy utilizes the concept of mindfulness, or being aware of and attentive to the current situation and moods. DBT also teaches skills to control intense emotions, reduce self-destructive behaviors, and improve relationships. DBT differs from CBT in that it integrates traditional CBT elements with mindfulness, acceptance, and techniques to improve a person's ability to tolerate stress and control his or her emotions. DBT recognizes the dialectical tension between the need for acceptance and the need for change.

- **Schema-Focused Therapy:** This type of therapy combines elements of CBT with other forms of psychotherapy that focus on reframing schemas, or the ways people view themselves. This approach is based on the idea that BPD stems from a dysfunctional self-image—possibly brought on by negative childhood experiences—that affects how people react to their environment, interact with others, and cope with problems or stress.

- **Systems Training for Emotional Predictability and Problem Solving (STEPPS):** This is a type of group therapy that aims to educate family members, significant others, and healthcare professionals about BPD and gives them guidance on how to interact consistently with the person with the disorder using the STEPPS approach and terminology. STEPPS is designed to supplement other treatments the patient may be receiving, such as medication or individual psychotherapy.

Families of people with BPD may also benefit from therapy. The challenges of dealing with a loved one with BPD on a daily basis can be very stressful, and family members may unknowingly act in ways that worsen their relative's symptoms. Some therapies include family members in treatment sessions. These types of programs help families develop skills to better understand and support a relative with BPD. Other therapies focus on the needs of family members and help them understand the obstacles and strategies for caring for a loved one with BPD.

Other types of psychotherapy may be helpful for some people with BPD. Therapists often adapt psychotherapy to better meet a person's needs. Therapists may also switch from one type of psychotherapy to another, mix techniques from different therapies, or use a combination of psychotherapies.

Medications

Medications should not be used as the primary treatment for BPD as the benefits are unclear. However, in some cases, a mental health professional may recommend medications to treat specific symptoms, such as mood swings, depression, or other disorders that may occur with BPD.

Treatment with medications may require care from more than one medical professional. Because of the high risk of suicide among people with BPD, healthcare providers should exercise caution when prescribing medications that may be lethal in the event of an overdose. Certain medications can cause different side effects in different people. Talk to your doctor about what to expect from a particular medication.

Other Treatments

Some people with BPD experience severe symptoms and require intensive, often inpatient, care. Others may use some outpatient treatments but never need hospitalization or emergency care. Although in rare cases, some people who develop this disorder may improve without any treatment, most people benefit from and improve their quality of life by seeking treatment.

How Can I Help A Friend Or Relative Who Has BPD?

If you know someone who has BPD, it affects you too. The first and most important thing you can do is help your friend or relative get the right diagnosis and treatment. You may need to make an appointment and go with your friend or relative to see the doctor. Encourage him or her to stay in treatment or to seek different treatment if symptoms do not appear to improve with the current treatment.

To help a friend or relative you can:

- Offer emotional support, understanding, patience, and encouragement—change can be difficult and frightening to people with BPD, but it is possible for them to get better over time.

- Learn about mental disorders, including BPD, so you can understand what your friend or relative is experiencing.

- With written permission from your friend or loved one, talk with his or her therapist to learn about therapies that may involve family members. Alternatively, you can encourage your loved one who is in treatment for BPD to ask about family therapy.

- Seek counseling from your own therapist about helping a loved one with BPD. It should not be the same therapist that your loved one with BPD is seeing.

Never ignore comments about someone's intent or plan to harm himself or herself or someone else. Report such comments to the person's therapist or doctor. In urgent or potentially life-threatening situations, you may need to call the police or dial 911.

How Can I Help Myself If I Have BPD?

Although it may take some time, you can get better with treatment. To help yourself:

- Talk to your doctor about treatment options and stick with treatment.

- Try to maintain a stable schedule of meals and sleep times.

- Engage in mild activity or exercise to help reduce stress.

- Set realistic goals for yourself.

- Break up large tasks into small ones, set some priorities, and do what you can, as you can.

- Try to spend time with other people and confide in a trusted friend or family member.

- Tell others about events or situations that may trigger symptoms.

- Expect your symptoms to improve gradually over time, not immediately. Be patient.

- Identify and seek out comforting situations, places, and people.

- Continue to educate yourself about this disorder.

- Don't drink alcohol or use illicit drugs—they will likely make things worse

Chapter 21

Histrionic Personality Disorder

What Is Histrionic Personality Disorder?

The term histrionic means "theatrical" or "dramatic." People with histrionic personality disorder have a compelling desire to be the center of attention at all times. To gain that attention, histrionics act in an extremely self-centered way. For example they may try to dominate conversations by interrupting others, behaving dramatically, and inappropriately. Or, they may dress provocatively and act seductively in inappropriate situations to gain the attention they seek. However, patients who suffer from the disorder possess a distorted image of themselves and lack a true feeling of self-worth, needing to derive their self-esteem from the approval of from others.

What Causes Histrionic Personality Disorder?

The definite cause of histrionic personality disorder remains unknown. However, a variety of hereditary and learned factors are believed to play a role. The disorder runs in families, which is suggestive of a genetic link, though a child could simply be repeating the behavior of a parent. Inconsistent parenting that leads to confusion in the child about acceptable behavior is another possible factor.

What Are The Symptoms Of Histrionic Personality Disorder?

The following symptoms are seen in people with histrionic personality disorder:

"Histrionic Personality Disorder," © 2017 Omnigraphics. Reviewed July 2017.

- Feeling uncomfortable if they are not the center of attention

- Self-centeredness to the point of being rash with others

- Rapid change in emotional states

- Behaving dramatically and exhibiting exaggerated emotions and expressions

- Giving excessive importance to physical appearance

- Dressing provocatively and looking seductive

- Shifting blame to others for failure or disappointment

- Sensitivity to disapproval or criticism

- Acting rashly without thinking rationally

- Approaches relationships in a shallow and fake manner

- Dislike towards routine, often starting projects and leaving them incomplete or skipping them all together

- Seeks approval and reassurance of others

- Being gullible and easily influenced by others

- Easily frustrated and seeks instant gratification

How Is Histrionic Personality Disorder Diagnosed?

Once doctors identify the symptoms, they carry out a physical examination and review the patient's complete medical history. Laboratory tests or imaging tests may also be done to rule out any possible physical causes. The patient will then be referred to a psychiatrist or psychologist who will diagnose the disorder based on a psychological evaluation. The patient's behavior, overall appearance, and psychological profile are considered during diagnosis. Patients suffering from histrionic personality disorder often also suffer from depression or anxiety, leading them to seek out professional help.

How Is Histrionic Personality Disorder Treated?

Talk therapy, otherwise known as psychotherapy, is the preferred treatment for histrionic personality disorder. The goal of talk therapy is to help patients recognize the motivations behind their thinking and behavior and to, in turn, approach the individuals around them in a positive and productive manner. However, treating patients with the disorder can be challenging since they often believe that they do not need treatment and can despise routine. In the case of depression that co-occurs with the disorder, antidepressants are prescribed, but generally not for extended durations.

What Complications Exist For Histrionic Personality Disorder?

The disorder will often affect the patient's social and romantic relationships. Patients with histrionic personality disorder are also at a higher risk of suffering from depression compared to the general population.

Can Histrionic Personality Disorder Be Prevented?

Though the disorder cannot be prevented, people who are prone to the condition can be equipped with techniques to deal with situations in a more constructive manner.

What Is The Outlook For The Disorder?

Most people with histrionic personality disorder lead productive lives and integrate with society in the long run. However, people with severe symptoms are likely to face significant problems in day-to-day life without ongoing treatment.

References

1. "Histrionic Personality Disorder," Cleveland Clinic, March 4, 2014.

2. "Histrionic Personality Disorder," Counselling Directory, 2017.

3. Berger, Fred K., MD. "Histrionic Personality Disorder," University of Iowa Stead Family Children's Hospital, November 18, 2016.

Chapter 22

Factitious Disorders

Difficult to diagnose and treat, factitious disorder is a rare mental disorder in which an individual acts as though they are sick when in reality they are mimicking or intentionally creating the symptoms of a disease or condition. Patients with factitious disorder may lie about symptoms, bring about symptoms by self-injury, needlessly under painful diagnostic procedures, and tamper with the results of the medical tests. Unlike those who lie about medical conditions for monetary gain or other compensation, the only goal of those with factitious disorder is to receive sympathy and special attention from family, friends, and the medical community. Factitious disorder is associated with preexisting mental illnesses such as depression and anxiety as well as stressful living conditions.

Factitious disorder can be subdivided into two types. The first is referred to factitious disorder imposed on self (in the past this subtype was referred to as Munchausen syndrome after the 18th Century German figure who regularly exaggerated his exploits). The person affected will themselves mimic a mental or physical illness. For example the person will appear confused, making absurd statements, and say they are hallucinating. They may also bring about physical symptoms such as stomach pains or seizures. The second type is factitious disorder imposed on others (previously referred to as Munchausen by proxy). In this manifestation, the person will impose false physical or psychological symptoms on another person. This is usually seen with a parent falsely presenting their child as sick, often putting the child at serious risk of harm as the result of unnecessary tests or medical procedures.

"Factitious Disorders," © 2017 Omnigraphics. Reviewed July 2017.

What Are The Symptoms?

The symptoms of factitious disorder are difficult to identify as the person can go to great lengths to hide their deception. Warning signs usually involve mimicking or exaggerating sickness or injury as well as:

- Episodes of lying.

- Self-injury—Individuals may inject themselves with harmful bacteria, milk, or feces to bring about symptoms or physically injure themselves by cutting or burning.

- Tampering with the results of diagnostic tests by such actions as manipulating medical instruments or contaminating urine samples with blood.

- Using aliases in order to visit a range of medical facilities and doctors.

- Persistent symptoms even after appropriate treatment.

- Extensive and specialized knowledge of medical conditions, tests, and treatment procedures.

- Repeated hospital stays.

- Unwillingness to allow the healthcare professionals to talk to their family and friends.

- Unwillingness to submit to psychiatric evaluation.

What Are The Causes Of Factitious Disorder?

The cause of factitious disorder is unknown, but researchers have found a strong link to preexisting behavioral and psychological issues along with stressful living conditions.

There may be several possible risk factors associated with factitious disorder. Research suggests that a childhood trauma in the form of physical, verbal, or emotional abuse as well as neglect can be a major factor. This can lead to poor sense of self or a loss of identity. Loss of a loved one that leads to a persistent sense of abandonment can also be a factor as well as past experiences of hospital stays that attracted significant attention from family and others. This condition can occasionally be seen in healthcare workers.

Diagnosis

Diagnosing factitious disorder is challenging given the amount of misinformation provided by the patient. Medical professionals first must gather as much of an accurate medical history as possible despite the exaggerations, misdirection, and potential use of aliases during treatment. They must then also rule out any possible physical or alternate mental condition (such as psychosis), which requires a thorough review of medical tests, imagery, and lab work. Interviewing the patient and observing his or her behavior is also key to diagnosing the condition. The patient may overdramatize his or symptoms, may present information that contradicts previous medical findings or the recollections of their caregivers, and may appear over eager to submit to painful or invasive tests. Medical professionals will then compare their findings to the criteria for factitious disorder as outlined in *Diagnostic and Statistical Manual of Mental Disorder*, Fifth Edition (DSM-5), published by the American Psychiatric Association (APA).

Treatment

No standard protocols or therapies are currently available for treatment of factitious disorders. However, it has been found that the affected person will respond better to a nonjudgmental approach. With this kind of approach, they may be more willing to be treated by a mental health professional. Also, having a primary care physician, or other medical professional act as a gatekeeper who monitors all medical care of a patient, is the key to accomplishing the first goal of treatment, which is to end or reduce that person's misuse of the medical system.

Psychotherapy will help in coping with underlying issues including stress and depression. Medications for preexisting mental health disorders may be used. If the disorder is found to be serious, extensive hospital stay and treatment may be required.

References

1. "An Overview Of Factitious Disorders," Cleveland Clinic, March 28, 2017.

2. "Factitious Disorder," Mayo Clinic, May 31, 2017.

Chapter 23

Delusional Disorder

What Is Delusional Disorder?

A delusion is a mistaken impression maintained by an individual that is contradictory to reality or plausible explanation. Persons with delusional disorder (DD) have untrue beliefs that persist for more than a month's duration. Some delusions that patients experience cannot be explained, but some of them could be realistic, lead to the disorder remaining undiagnosed. Delusional disorder, previously known as paranoid disorder, is classified under psychotic illnesses. People with delusional disorder perceive things differently and misinterpret experiences.

Delusional disorder differs from other psychotic disorders with respect to how people carry on with their daily lives. People with more common psychotic disorders, such as schizophrenia, become so preoccupied with their delusions that it hampers their daily routine. Those with delusional disorder, on the other hand, function normally in society. They remain employed, perform daily tasks without hindrance, and do not act bizarrely. The incidence of delusional disorder in the general population is rare. The disorder occurs in middle to late adulthood and occurs more in women than men.

What Are The Symptoms And Subtypes Of Delusional Disorder?

The dominant or only symptom of delusional disorder is delusions. While delusions are prominent in other psychotic disorders such as schizophrenia and bipolar disorder, the absence of accompanying symptoms such as hallucinations, mood swings, disorganized thinking, and

"Delusional Disorder," © 2017 Omnigraphics. Reviewed July 2017.

cognitive deficits are used to make the diagnosis of delusional disorder. Early signs of illness may include a basic mistrust with people, unwarranted jealousy of spouse, or preoccupation with loyalty in relation to friends and relatives. The person is also overly sensitive to harmless remarks or perceived slights and tends to hold a long-standing grudge toward the subject of their delusion despite evidence to the contrary.

Some of the recognized subtypes of delusional disorder are:

- **Erotomania:** Implausible belief held by the affected person that another person is in love him or her. The person believed to be in love with the delusional person can be a famous person or a total stranger. Those suffering from this type of delusional disorder will often try to establish contact with the object of their fixation through letters, telephone calls, and surveillance is seen. This may be tantamount to stalking and may have legal implications.

- **Jealous type:** Delusional belief that his or her spouse (or sexual partner) is unfaithful. Also known as conjugal paranoia, or Othello syndrome, the affected person justifies his or her conviction on the basis of false conclusions despite the lack of objective evidence. Physical violence may or may not accompany this subtype.

- **Grandiose type:** Also called megalomania, this type is characterized by exaggerated beliefs of grandeur and self-worth as well as extreme arrogance. The affected person believes he is omnipotent, famous, and powerful and the delusions typically have a religious, fictional, or supernatural content.

- **Persecutory:** Persistent conviction that he or she is being plotted against, maligned, or harassed with intent to cause harm. The delusional person may relentlessly seek legal recourse through courts and law enforcement agencies and may even resort to violence in retaliation for the perceived threat.

- **Somatic:** Characterized by intense preoccupation with imagined defects in physical appearance (body dysmorphic disorder) and bodily function (hypochondriasis), which focuses on imagined illnesses/disorders contrary to medical evidence. This type may also include delusional infestation (DI) in which the affected persons hold a rigid belief that they are infested with parasites or pathogens and patients may typically describe sensations of "crawling" and "biting" to substantiate their beliefs.

How Is Delusional Disorder Diagnosed?

Delusional disorder is diagnosed on the basis of a thorough psychological assessment. A physical examination and diagnostic tests, including imaging tests and blood tests, are carried out to rule out other causes. Interviews with family members and friends to understand past history and behavioral symptoms are important tools that assist in diagnosis. Non-bizarre delusions persisting for more than a month and absence of symptoms related to schizophrenia and other psychotic disorders lead to confirmation of diagnosis. The doctor will also assess if the person will likely act on delusions.

What Causes Delusional Disorder?

The causes and triggers for delusional disorder are not known in medical circles. But the following factors are thought to play a role.

- **Genetics:** The disorder is seen in families that have a history of schizophrenia and delusional disorder suggesting a genetic link. The disorder might be inherited from parents to their children hereditarily.

- **Environmental or psychological:** There is evidence that suggests that the disorder may develop as a result of stress. Substance abuse such as alcoholism and drug abuse could lead to the disorder. Remaining in isolation is also a risk factor. The disorder has been identified in refugees particularly in people with low sight and hearing leading to the observation.

- **Biological:** Researchers are investigating anomalies in the brain that could be a contributing factor for the disorder. Defects in regions of the brain that control perception and thinking may be linked to the disorder.

What Is The Treatment For Delusional Disorder?

A combination of psychotherapy and medication is used to treat delusional disorder. Denial about delusions, poor insight, and refusal to seek help are deterrents to treatment. Establishing a good rapport between doctor and patient is crucial to successful treatment. Medications help in recovery to some extent. Medications commonly used for treatment include conventional antipsychotics (neuroleptics), atypical antipsychotics, tranquilizers, and antidepressants. Psychotherapy is also recommended and therapy types such as cognitive behavior therapy, family therapy, and individual counseling help the person manage stress and the impact of delusions in daily functioning.

What Are The Complications That Arise Due To Delusional Disorder?

Delusions could lead to depression because of difficulties that arise out of such thinking. Persons who act on their delusions may become violent and get into legal difficulties. If the delusions are severe, then people could become alienated from family and friends.

What Is The Outlook For Recovery?

The outlook for recovery depends on factors such as the type of delusional disorder, life circumstances, what support is available for the person, and his or her willingness to remain under treatment. Delusional disorder is a chronic condition with chances of complete recovery. Some patients experience periods that are free of incidents mixed with episodes of delusions. Most patients with delusional disorder do not seek help because of fear or embarrassment. If treatment is not sought, delusional disorder becomes a lifelong affliction.

Is Delusional Disorder Preventable?

Prevention strategies do not exist currently for delusional disorder but the effect of illness can be minimized with treatment, and the patient can lead a productive life in the company of family and friends.

References

1. "Delusional Disorder And Substance Abuse," American Addiction Centers, n.d.

2. "Treatments For Delusional Disorder," Cochrane, n.d.

3. "Delusional Disorder As A Partial Psychosis," U.S. National Library of Medicine (NLM), National Institutes of Health (NIH), 2014.

4. "Understanding Delusions," U.S. National Library of Medicine (NLM), National Institutes of Health (NIH), 2009.

5. Schulz, Charles "Delusional Disorder," Merck Manual, n.d.

6. "Mental Health And Delusional Disorder," WebMD, n.d.

Chapter 24

Dissociative Disorders

Dissociation is a psychological state that involves feeling disconnected from reality. A dissociative disorder is a mental health condition in which the affected person experiences a disconnection from their thoughts, feelings, memories, perceptions, consciousness, or identity.

For many people, dissociation is used as a defense mechanism to block out the memory of extremely stressful or traumatic life experiences, particularly from childhood. Dissociative disorders are often found in individuals who were exposed to physical, emotional, or sexual abuse as children, for instance, and in those who endured such traumatic events as natural disasters, wars, accidents, violent crimes, or the tragic loss of a loved one. Dissociative disorders often manifest themselves during stressful situations in adulthood, which can make it difficult for people affected to deal with the challenges of everyday life.

Research suggests that around 2 to 3 percent of people are affected by dissociative disorders. Some of the common symptoms include episodes of memory or sensory loss, feelings of emotional detachment, or a sense of watching oneself from the outside. Dissociative disorders

Dissociative Disorder

A person with dissociative disorder would have greater exaggeration and rigidity of parts with little internal communication. A person with dissociative disorder has more encapsulated parts of self, frozen in traumatic experience and a concomitant sense of self-injury, defectiveness and badness than do most other people.

"Dissociative Disorders," © 2017 Omnigraphics. Reviewed July 2017.

Their behavior is therefore considered by others as "borderline like" or "crazy," but in actuality, is highly rational and predictable once the trauma-organized system is understood.

(Source: "Post-Traumatic Stress, Sexual Trauma And Dissociative Disorder: Issues Related To Intimacy And Sexuality," National Institute of Justice (NIJ), U.S. Department of Justice (DOJ).)

often coincide with other mental health issues, such as mood swings, attention deficits, drug and alcohol dependence, anxiety, panic attacks, and suicidal tendencies.

According to the American Psychiatric Association's *Diagnostic and Statistical Manual of Mental Disorders (DSM)*, dissociative disorders take three main forms: depersonalization/derealization disorder; dissociative amnesia; and dissociative identity disorder.

Depersonalization/Derealization Disorder

Depersonalization is a profound sense of detachment or alienation from one's own body, mind, or identity. People with depersonalization disorder may experience an "out of body" sensation, or feel as if they are looking at their own life from an external perspective, like watching a movie. Some people affected by this condition may not recognize their own face in a mirror.

Derealization is the sense that the world does not seem real. People with derealization disorder may report that their surroundings appear hazy, foggy, phony, or far away. Familiar places may seem unfamiliar, and close friends may seem like strangers. In some cases, situations take on a dreamlike quality, and the affected person may feel disoriented and have difficulty determining what is real and what is not.

Dissociative Amnesia

Dissociative amnesia is the inability to remember people, events, or personal information. This memory loss is too substantial to be considered normal forgetfulness, and it is not related to aging, disease, or a head injury. In most cases, people with dissociative amnesia forget a traumatic incident or an extremely stressful period of time. They may also experience smaller lapses in which they forget the content of a conversation or a talent or skill that they have learned.

Dissociative amnesia may be localized, selective, or generalized. In localized amnesia, the memory lapse is concerned with a particular event or span of time. In selective amnesia, the affected person forgets certain parts of a traumatic incident but may remember others.

In generalized amnesia, the affected person is unable to remember anything about their own identity or life history. In rare cases dissociative amnesia may take the form of fugue, in which a person travels for hours or days without a sense of their own identity, then suddenly regains awareness and wonders how they got there.

Dissociative Identity Disorder

Dissociative identity disorder, formerly known as multiple personality disorder, is characterized by a deep uncertainty or confusion about one's identity. People affected by this disorder may feel the presence of other people or alternate identities (known as "alters") within themselves.

Each of these alters may have their own name, history, voice, mannerisms, and worldview.

A child who has suffered a severe psychological trauma is more likely to develop a dissociative identity disorder. Since the child's mind lacks the coping mechanisms to process the stressful experience, the still-developing personality may find it easier to dissociate and pretend that it was happening to someone else.

Treatment For Dissociative Disorders

Before diagnosing a dissociative disorder, a doctor may perform tests to rule out physical conditions that may cause similar symptoms, such as a head injury, brain tumor, sleep deprivation, or drug addiction. If no physical cause is found, the patient may be referred to a mental health professional for further evaluation. The mental health specialist will likely inquire about childhood trauma and screen the patient for trauma-related conditions, such as anxiety, depression, posttraumatic stress disorder, and substance abuse. Although there is no medication to treat dissociation, antidepressants and anti-anxiety drugs may provide some relief from the symptoms of associated conditions.

Psychiatrists often treat dissociative disorders with counseling designed to help the patient cope with the underlying trauma. They view dissociation as a normal defense mechanism that the brain may use to adapt to a difficult situation in early life. Dissociation only becomes dysfunctional when it persists into adulthood and governs an individual's response to everyday challenges. In these cases, the patient may benefit from a course of psychotherapy to help them understand and process the traumatic event.

Eye movement desensitization and reprocessing (EMDR) is another technique that can help alleviate symptoms related to psychological trauma. In EMDR, the patient makes side to side eye motions, usually by following the movement of the therapist's finger, while recalling the traumatic incident. Although doctors are not sure how EMDR works, it appears to help the brain process distressing memories so that they have less impact on the patient's daily life.

References

1. "Dissociative Disorders," National Alliance on Mental Illness, n.d.

2. "Dissociative Disorders," NHS Choices, Gov.UK, 2014.

3. "Dissociation FAQs," International Society for the Study of Trauma and Dissociation, 2014.

Chapter 25

Psychosis

What Is Psychosis?

The word psychosis is used to describe conditions that affect the mind, where there has been some loss of contact with reality. When someone becomes ill in this way it is called a psychotic episode. During a period of psychosis, a person's thoughts and perceptions are disturbed and the individual may have difficulty understanding what is real and what is not.

Psychotic Disorders

Psychotic disorders are characterized by dysregulation of thought processes. In particular, schizophrenia has hallmark symptoms of delusions—which are false beliefs—and hallucinations—which are hearing and/or seeing sensory information which is not actually present and is not apparent to others. Schizoaffective disorder is a disorder in which, as its name implies, individuals have features of both schizophrenia and mood disorders. Typically, psychotic disorders are treated with antipsychotic medications and some forms of psychosocial interventions.

(Source: "Psychotic Disorders," Centers for Disease Control and Prevention (CDC).)

What Are The Symptoms Of Psychosis?

Symptoms of psychosis include delusions (false beliefs) and hallucinations (seeing or hearing things that others do not see or hear). Other symptoms include incoherent or nonsense speech, and behavior that is inappropriate for the situation. A person in a psychotic episode

---

About This Chapter: This chapter includes text excerpted from "Recovery After An Initial Schizophrenia Episode (RAISE)—RAISE Questions And Answers," National Institute of Mental Health (NIMH), October 7, 2015.

may also experience depression, anxiety, sleep problems, social withdrawal, lack of motivation, and difficulty functioning overall.

What Causes Psychosis?

There is not one specific cause of psychosis. Psychosis may be a symptom of a mental illness, such as schizophrenia or bipolar disorder, but there are other causes, as well. Sleep deprivation, some general medical conditions, certain prescription medications, and the abuse of alcohol or other drugs, such as marijuana, can cause psychotic symptoms. Because there are many different causes of psychosis, it is important to see a qualified healthcare professional (e.g., psychologist, psychiatrist, or trained social worker) in order to receive a thorough assessment and accurate diagnosis. A mental illness, such as schizophrenia, is typically diagnosed by excluding all of these other causes of psychosis.

How Common Is Psychosis?

Approximately 3 percent of the people in the United States (3 out of 100 people) will experience psychosis at some time in their lives. About 100,000 adolescents and young adults in the United States experience first episode psychosis each year.

What Are The Early Warning Signs Of Psychosis?

Typically, a person will show changes in their behavior before psychosis develops. The list below includes behavioral warning signs for psychosis.

- Worrisome drop in grades or job performance

- New trouble thinking clearly or concentrating

- Suspiciousness, paranoid ideas, or uneasiness with others

- Withdrawing socially, spending a lot more time alone than usual

- Unusual, overly intense new ideas, strange feelings, or having no feelings at all

- Decline in self-care or personal hygiene

- Difficulty telling reality from fantasy

- Confused speech or trouble communicating

Any one of these items by itself may not be significant, but someone with several of the items on the list should consult a mental health professional. A qualified psychologist, psychiatrist, or trained social worker will be able to make a diagnosis and help develop a treatment plan. Early treatment of psychosis increases the chance of a successful recovery. If you notice these changes in behavior and they begin to intensify or do not go away, it is important to seek help.

Do People Recover From Psychosis?

With early diagnosis and appropriate treatment, it is possible to recover from psychosis. Many people who receive early treatment never have another psychotic episode. For other people, recovery means the ability to live a fulfilling and productive life, even if psychotic symptoms return sometimes.

What Should I Do If I Think Someone Is Having A Psychotic Episode?

If you think someone you know is experiencing psychosis, encourage the person to seek treatment as early as possible. Psychosis can be treated effectively, and early intervention increases the chance of a successful outcome. To find a qualified treatment program, contact your healthcare professional. If someone having a psychotic episode is in distress or you are concerned about their safety, consider taking them to the nearest emergency room, or calling 911.

Why Is Early Treatment Important?

Left untreated, psychotic symptoms can lead to disruptions in school and work, strained family relations, and separation from friends. The longer the symptoms go untreated, the greater the risk of additional problems. These problems can include substance abuse, going to the emergency department, being admitted to the hospital, having legal trouble, or becoming homeless.

Studies have shown that many people experiencing first episode psychosis in the United States typically have symptoms for more than a year before receiving treatment. It is important to reduce this duration of untreated psychosis because people tend to do better when they receive effective treatment as early as possible.

What Is Shared Decision Making And How Does It Work In Early Treatment?

Shared decision making means individuals and their healthcare providers work together to find the best treatment options based on the individual's unique needs and preferences.

Clients, treatment-team members, and (when appropriate) relatives are active participants in the process.

What Is The Role Of Medication In Treatment?

Antipsychotic medications help reduce psychotic symptoms. Like medications for any illness, antipsychotic drugs have benefits and risks. Individuals should talk with their healthcare providers about the benefits of taking antipsychotic medication as well as potential side effects, dosage, and preferences like taking a daily pill or a monthly injection.

What Is Supported Employment/Education (SEE) And Why Is It Important?

For young adults, psychosis can hurt school attendance and academic performance or make it difficult to find or keep a job. Supported Employment/Education (SEE) is one way to help individuals return to work or school. A SEE specialist helps clients develop the skills they need to achieve school and work goals. In addition, the specialist can be a bridge between clients and educators or employers. SEE services are an important part of coordinated specialty care and are valued by many clients. Findings from RAISE-IES showed that SEE services often brought people into care and engaged them in treatment because it directly addressed their personal goals.

Chapter 26

Schizophrenia

Schizophrenia is a chronic and severe mental disorder that affects how a person thinks, feels, and behaves. People with schizophrenia may seem like they have lost touch with reality. Although schizophrenia is not as common as other mental disorders, the symptoms can be very disabling.

Schizophrenia is a severe, lifelong brain disorder. People who have it may hear voices, see things that aren't there or believe that others are reading or controlling their minds. In men, symptoms usually start in the late teens and early 20s. They include hallucinations, or seeing things, and delusions such as hearing voices. For women, they start in the mid-20s to early 30s. Other symptoms include:

- Unusual thoughts or perceptions
- Disorders of movement
- Difficulty speaking and expressing emotion
- Problems with attention, memory and organization

No one is sure what causes schizophrenia, but your genetic makeup and brain chemistry probably play a role. Medicines can relieve many of the symptoms, but it can take several tries before you find the right drug. You can reduce relapses by staying on your medicine for as long as your doctor recommends. With treatment, many people improve enough to lead satisfying lives.

(Source: "Schizophrenia," MentalHealth.gov, U.S. Department of Health and Human Services (HHS).)

About This Chapter: This chapter includes text excerpted from "Schizophrenia," National Institute of Mental Health (NIMH), February 2016.

Signs And Symptoms Of Schizophrenia

Symptoms of schizophrenia usually start between ages 16 and 30. In rare cases, children have schizophrenia too.

The symptoms of schizophrenia fall into three categories: positive, negative, and cognitive.

Positive symptoms: "Positive" symptoms are psychotic behaviors not generally seen in healthy people. People with positive symptoms may "lose touch" with some aspects of reality. Symptoms include:

- Hallucinations

- Delusions

- Thought disorders (unusual or dysfunctional ways of thinking)

- Movement disorders (agitated body movements)

Negative symptoms: "Negative" symptoms are associated with disruptions to normal emotions and behaviors. Symptoms include:

- "Flat affect" (reduced expression of emotions via facial expression or voice tone)

- Reduced feelings of pleasure in everyday life

- Difficulty beginning and sustaining activities

- Reduced speaking

Cognitive symptoms: For some patients, the cognitive symptoms of schizophrenia are subtle, but for others, they are more severe and patients may notice changes in their memory or other aspects of thinking. Symptoms include:

- Poor "executive functioning" (the ability to understand information and use it to make decisions)

- Trouble focusing or paying attention

- Problems with "working memory" (the ability to use information immediately after learning it)

Risk Factors Of Schizophrenia

There are several factors that contribute to the risk of developing schizophrenia.

Genes and environment: Scientists have long known that schizophrenia sometimes runs in families. However, there are many people who have schizophrenia who don't have a family member with the disorder and conversely, many people with one or more family members with the disorder who do not develop it themselves.

Scientists believe that many different genes may increase the risk of schizophrenia, but that no single gene causes the disorder by itself. It is not yet possible to use genetic information to predict who will develop schizophrenia.

Scientists also think that interactions between genes and aspects of the individual's environment are necessary for schizophrenia to develop. Environmental factors may involve:

- Exposure to viruses

- Malnutrition before birth

- Problems during birth

- Psychosocial factors

Different brain chemistry and structure: Scientists think that an imbalance in the complex, interrelated chemical reactions of the brain involving the neurotransmitters (substances that brain cells use to communicate with each other) dopamine and glutamate, and possibly others, plays a role in schizophrenia.

Some experts also think problems during brain development before birth may lead to faulty connections. The brain also undergoes major changes during puberty, and these changes could trigger psychotic symptoms in people who are vulnerable due to genetics or brain differences.

Treatments And Therapies For Schizophrenia

Because the causes of schizophrenia are still unknown, treatments focus on eliminating the symptoms of the disease. Treatments include:

Antipsychotics

Antipsychotic medications are usually taken daily in pill or liquid form. Some antipsychotics are injections that are given once or twice a month. Some people have side effects when they start taking medications, but most side effects go away after a few days. Doctors and patients can work together to find the best medication or medication combination, and the right dose.

Psychosocial Treatments

These treatments are helpful after patients and their doctor find a medication that works. Learning and using coping skills to address the everyday challenges of schizophrenia helps people to pursue their life goals, such as attending school or work. Individuals who participate in regular psychosocial treatment are less likely to have relapses or be hospitalized.

Coordinated Specialty Care (CSC)

This treatment model integrates medication, psychosocial therapies, case management, family involvement, and supported education and employment services, all aimed at reducing symptoms and improving quality of life.

How Can I Help Someone I Know With Schizophrenia?

Caring for and supporting a loved one with schizophrenia can be hard. It can be difficult to know how to respond to someone who makes strange or clearly false statements. It is important to understand that schizophrenia is a biological illness.

Here are some things you can do to help your loved one:

- Get them treatment and encourage them to stay in treatment

- Remember that their beliefs or hallucinations seem very real to them

- Tell them that you acknowledge that everyone has the right to see things their own way

- Be respectful, supportive, and kind without tolerating dangerous or inappropriate behavior

- Check to see if there are any support groups in your area

Chapter 27

Schizoaffective Disorder

What Is Schizoaffective Disorder?

Schizoaffective disorder is a chronic and treatable psychiatric illness. It is characterized by a combination of:

1. psychotic symptoms, such as those seen in schizophrenia and

2. mood symptoms, such as those seen in depression or bipolar disorder.

It is a psychiatric disorder that can affect a person's thinking, emotions, and behaviors and can impact all aspects of daily living, including work, school, social relationships, and self-care.

Schizoaffective disorder is considered a psychotic disorder because of its prominent features of hallucinations and delusions. Therefore, people with this illness have periods when they have difficulty understanding the reality around them. They may hear voices other people don't hear. They may have unusual thoughts and suspicions, such as believing that other people can read their minds, control their thoughts, or plot to harm them. These experiences can terrify people with the illness and make them withdraw and/or become agitated. Some individuals with this illness also lack expressiveness, have low motivation, are unable to experience pleasure, and do not show an interest in social relationships. In addition to these symptoms, nearly all people with schizoaffective disorder have some impairments in their memory, attention, and decision-making ability.

In addition to psychotic symptoms, individuals with schizoaffective disorder also experience mood episodes. While some people only experience symptoms of depression or mania,

About This Chapter: This chapter includes text excerpted from "What Is Schizoaffective Disorder?" U.S. Department of Veterans Affairs (VA), September 2016.

others experience both types of symptoms. The ups and downs experienced by someone with schizoaffective disorder are very different from the normal ups and downs that most people experience from time to time. Changes in mood can last for hours, days, weeks, or months. In between these extremes, the person's mood may be normal. Families and society are affected by schizoaffective disorder as well. Symptoms may result in poor social functioning and poor job or school performance. Many people with schizoaffective disorder have difficulty holding a job or caring for themselves, so they rely on others for help. There are treatments that help improve functioning and relieve many symptoms of schizoaffective disorder. Recovery is possible! A combination of helpful therapies, education in managing one's illness, and supports to provide assistance and encouragement can lead to experiencing fewer symptoms, improving relationships with other people, and achieving meaningful and fulfilling life goals.

Prevalence Of Schizoaffective Disorder

Although the exact prevalence of schizoaffective disorder is not clear, experts estimate that it ranges from 0.2–0.5 percent. Schizoaffective disorder is more common in woman than in men. Individuals with a first degree relative (e.g., parent or sibling) with schizophrenia, bipolar disorder, or schizoaffective disorder are at increased risk of developing schizoaffective disorder, compared to someone with no family history of these disorders.

Causes Of Schizoaffective Disorder

There is no simple answer to what causes schizoaffective disorder because several factors play a part in the onset of the disorder. These include a genetic or family history of schizoaffective disorder, schizophrenia, or bipolar disorder, biological factors, environmental stressors, and stressful life events. Research shows that the risk of schizoaffective disorder results from the influence of genes acting together with biological and environmental factors. A family history of schizoaffective disorder does not necessarily mean children or other relatives will develop the disorder.

However, studies have shown that schizoaffective disorder does run in families, and a family history of schizoaffective disorder, schizophrenia, or bipolar disorder is one of the strongest and most consistent risk factors for the disorder. In terms of biological factors, an imbalance of the neurotransmitters dopamine, glutamate, norepinephrine, and serotonin is also linked to schizoaffective disorder. Neurotransmitters are brain chemicals that communicate information throughout the brain and body. However, the exact role of these neurotransmitters in schizoaffective disorder is unclear.

In addition to genetic and biological factors, others believe that environment also plays a key role in whether someone will develop schizoaffective disorder. Some of the environmental factors believed to be linked to schizophrenia-spectrum disorders, including schizoaffective disorder, are malnutrition, maternal illness or exposure to toxins before birth, obstetric complications, poverty, and substance use. Cannabis use, especially before age 15, has also been identified as a risk factor in developing psychotic symptoms. Stressful life events, such as family conflict, early parental loss or separation, and physical or sexual abuse, are also associated with schizophrenia-spectrum disorders.

> Schizoaffective disorder usually begins in late adolescence or early adulthood, often between the ages of 16 and 30. The initial symptoms of the disorder can vary greatly the onset of psychotic symptoms may be abrupt or gradual, and they might present before or after the onset of mood symptoms. Schizoaffective disorder with manic symptoms appears to be more common in young adults, while schizoaffective disorder with depressive symptoms alone appears to be more common in older adults.
>
> The course of schizoaffective disorder over time varies considerably and may require hospitalization. Most people experience periods of symptom exacerbation and remission, while others are more chronically ill and maintain a steady level of moderate to severe symptoms and disability over time. Some individuals have a milder course of the illness. Although the disorder is often life long, symptoms tend to improve over the person's life.

Symptoms Of Schizoaffective Disorder

A person with schizoaffective disorder experiences mood symptoms at the same time they experience psychotic symptoms, but they also experience psychotic symptoms even during periods in which their mood is relatively normal. The person will be diagnosed with either schizoaffective disorder (depressive type) or schizoaffective disorder (bipolar type). The depressive type is diagnosed in those who have experienced a major depressive episode only with no history of mania. The bipolar type is diagnosed in those who have experienced a manic episode during the course of their illness. A major depressive episode also may have occurred, but it is not required for this subtype. This handout describes psychotic, mood, and cognitive symptoms that are seen in schizoaffective disorder. To be diagnosed with schizoaffective disorder, the symptoms a person experiences must be severe enough to impair social, work, or other areas of functioning.

Psychotic Symptoms

The symptoms of psychotic disorders are generally categorized as positive symptoms or negative symptoms. Positive symptoms refer to thoughts, perceptions, and behaviors that are present in people with psychotic disorders but are ordinarily absent in other people. They include symptoms such as hallucinations and delusions. These symptoms can come and go. Sometimes they are severe, and sometimes they are hardly noticeable. Conversely, negative symptoms are the absence of thoughts, perceptions, or behaviors that are ordinarily present in other people. These symptoms are often stable throughout much of a person's life.

- **Hallucinations** are false perceptions. A person may hear, see, feel, smell, or taste things that are not actually there.

- **Delusions** are false beliefs that are held in spite of overwhelming evidence against them.

- **Disorganized thinking and speech** is when a person has trouble organizing his or her thoughts or connecting them logically. They may string words together in an incoherent way that is hard to understand, often referred to as a "word salad." The person may make "loose associations," where they rapidly shift from one topic to an unrelated topic, making it very difficult to follow their conversation.

- **Grossly disorganized behavior or catatonic behavior.** Disorganized behaviors include bizarre behaviors, unpredictable or inappropriate responses, and lack of inhibition or impulse control.

- **Negative symptoms** are the absence of thoughts, perceptions, or behaviors that are ordinarily present in other people.

Depressive Symptoms

In schizoaffective disorder, a depressive episode is a period during which a person feels depressed most of the day, nearly every day, for at least two weeks. The person must also experience at least four of these symptoms:

- Loss of interest or pleasure in things once found to be enjoyable

- Significant weight loss when not dieting, weight gain, or a decrease or increase in appetite

- Insomnia or hypersomnia (difficulty falling asleep or staying asleep, waking early in the morning and not being able to get back to sleep, or sleeping excessively)

- Psychomotor agitation (e.g., inability to sit still or pacing) or psychomotor retardation (e.g., slowed speech, thinking, and body movements)

- Fatigue or loss of energy

- Feelings of worthlessness or excessive or inappropriate guilt

- Decreased ability to think or concentrate, or indecisiveness

- Recurrent thoughts of death (not just fear of dying), recurrent suicidal ideation without a specific plan, a specific plan for committing suicide, or a suicide attempt

Manic Symptoms

A manic episode is a period during which a person feels extremely happy or irritable and has increased energy most of the day, nearly every day, for at least one week (less if hospitalized). The person must also experience at least three of these symptoms (four if the mood is only irritable):

- Inflated self-esteem or grandiosity (has a high opinion of self and may be unrealistic about their abilities)

- Decreased need for sleep (e.g., feels rested after only 3 hours of sleep)

- More talkative than usual or pressure to keep talking

- Flight of ideas or racing thoughts (has too many thoughts at the same time or rapid speech that jumps from topic to topic)

- Distractibility (attention is easily drawn to unimportant or irrelevant things)

- Increased goal-directed activities (e.g., social, sexual, or at work or school) or psychomotor agitation (purposeless nongoal-directed activity)

- Excessive involvement in activities with a high potential for painful consequences (e.g., shopping sprees, driving recklessly, and unsafe sex)

Cognitive Symptoms

Although cognitive symptoms are not part of the diagnosis for schizoaffective disorder, nearly all individuals with the disorder experience some cognitive impairment. Cognition refers to mental processes that allow us to perform day-to-day functions, such as the ability to pay attention, to remember, and to solve problems. Cognitive impairments are considered a core feature of schizoaffective disorder and contribute to difficulties in work, social relationships, and independent living.

Diagnosis Of Schizoaffective Disorder

Schizoaffective disorder is a psychiatric disorder that must be diagnosed by a trained mental health professional. Diagnostic interviews and medical evaluations are used to determine the diagnosis. There are currently no physical or lab tests that can diagnose schizoaffective disorder, but they can help rule out other medical or mental health conditions that sometimes have similar symptoms. To make the diagnosis, a trained mental health professional conducts a comprehensive interview and pays careful attention to the symptoms experienced, the severity of the symptoms, how long they have lasted, and which symptoms have overlapped in time.

The fact that this diagnosis includes features of both psychotic and mood disorders means that making an accurate diagnosis can be challenging. Individuals with schizoaffective disorder may be misdiagnosed with having another psychotic disorder, such as schizophrenia, schizophreniform disorder, brief psychotic disorder, or delusional disorder. Alternatively, they may be misdiagnosed with a mood disorder, such as major depression or bipolar disorder. The diagnosing clinician must also make sure symptoms are not due to a general medical condition and are not the direct result of drug use, medication, or toxin exposure. Therefore, a careful and thorough interview is needed to prevent misdiagnosis from occurring. It is useful to collect information from relatives and friends who have observed the individual's behaviors and moods.

How Family Members Can Help

The family environment is very important in the recovery of individuals with schizoaffective disorder. Even though the disorder can be a frustrating illness, family members can help the process of recovery in many ways.

Encourage Treatment And Rehabilitation

- The first step is to visit a doctor for a thorough evaluation. If possible, it is often helpful for family members to be present at the evaluation to offer support, help answer the doctor's questions, and learn about the illness.

- If medication is prescribed, family members can provide support in regularly taking those medications.

- Family members can help the person fit taking medication into their daily routine.

- Family members can be very helpful in supporting treatment attendance.

Provide Support

- Family stress can contribute to symptom relapses. Conversely, family support can help people cope with stress and decrease the risk of relapse.

- It is best if family members try to be understanding rather than critical, negative, or blaming. It may be difficult at times, but families often do best when they are patient and appreciate any progress that is being made, however slow it may be.

- Family members try to make sense of psychotic disorders by understanding its causes.

Take Care Of Themselves

- Family members often feel guilty about spending time away from their ill relative; however, it is important that they take good care of themselves.

- Family members should not allow their ill relative to monopolize their time.

- Spending time alone or with other family members and friends is important for their own well-being.

- Counseling can often help family and friends better cope with a loved one's illness. Family members should not feel responsible for solving their relative's problems themselves. They can't. They should get the help of a mental health professional if needed.

Treatment Of Schizoaffective Disorder

There are a variety of medications and therapies available to those suffering from schizoaffective disorder. Medications can help reduce symptoms and are recommended as the first-line treatment for schizoaffective disorder.

Psychoeducation

Psychoeducation provides individuals with information about their illness and the most effective ways of treating symptoms and preventing relapse.

Social Skills Training

Many people with schizoaffective disorder have difficulties with social skills. Social skills training (SST) aims to correct these deficits by teaching skills to help express emotion and communicate more effectively, so individuals are more likely to achieve their goals, develop relationships, and live independently.

Family-Based Services

Mental illness affects the whole family. Family services teach families to work together toward recovery. In family-based services, the family and clinician meet to discuss problems the family is experiencing.

Illness Self-Management

Components of illness self-management include psychoeducation, teaching coping skills to manage stress and symptoms, relapse prevention, and social skills training.

Cognitive Behavioral Therapy (CBT)

Cognitive behavioral therapy (CBT) is a blend of two therapies: cognitive therapy and behavioral therapy. Treating schizoaffective disorder with CBT is challenging, but research has shown that CBT, as an add-on to medication, can help a person better cope with their illness. CBT can be done one-on-one or in a group setting.

Cognitive therapy focuses on a person's thoughts and beliefs and how they influence a person's mood and actions. CBT aims to change a person's thinking to be more adaptive and healthy. CBT helps individuals learn how to identify maladaptive thoughts, logically challenge them, and replace them with more adaptive thoughts.

Behavioral therapy focuses on a person's actions and aims to change unhealthy behavior patterns. CBT is skill-oriented, and people learn techniques to cope with life's challenges.

Assertive Community Treatment (ACT)

Assertive community treatment (ACT) is an approach that is most effective for individuals with the greatest service needs, such as those with a history of multiple hospitalizations or those who are homeless. In ACT, the person receives treatment from an interdisciplinary team of usually 10 to 12 professionals, including case managers, a psychiatrist, several nurses and social workers, vocational specialists, substance abuse treatment specialists, and peer specialists.

Electroconvulsive Therapy (ECT)

Electroconvulsive therapy (ECT) is a procedure used to treat severe or life-threatening depression. It is used when other treatments such as psychotherapy and medications have not worked. Electrical currents are briefly sent to the brain through electrodes placed on the head. The electrical current can last up to eight seconds, producing a short seizure.

Medication: What You Should Know

Because schizoaffective disorder involves many kinds of symptoms, the treatment can be complex. You and your doctor have a lot of choices of medications, and it is hard to know which one may work best for you. It is also often the case that more than one medication is required to treat mood symptoms and symptoms affecting your thinking processes. Sometimes the medication you first try may not lead to improvements in symptoms. This is because each person's brain chemistry is unique; what works well for one person may not do as well for another. Be open to trying a different medication or combination of medications in order to find a good fit. Let your doctor know if your symptoms have not improved or have worsened, and do not give up searching for the right medication!

- There are different types of medications that are effective for schizoaffective disorder. These include antipsychotic medications, mood stabilizers, and antidepressant medications.

- Once you have responded to treatment, it is important to continue treatment. To prevent symptoms from coming back or worsening, do not abruptly stop taking your medications, even if you are feeling better. Stopping your medication can cause a relapse. Medication should only be stopped under your doctor's supervision. If you want to stop taking your medication, talk to your doctor about how to correctly stop them.

- Like all medications, medications prescribed for schizoaffective disorder can have side effects. Your doctor will discuss some common side effects with you. In many cases, they are mild and tend to diminish with time. Some people have few or no side effects, and the side effects people typically experience are tolerable and subside in a few days. Sometimes, common side effects can persist or become bothersome. If you experience such side effects, discuss them with your doctor and be sure to talk to them before making any decisions about discontinuing treatment.

- In rare cases, these medications can cause severe side effects. Contact your doctor immediately if you experience one or more severe symptoms.

Part Four
Behavioral, Impulse Control, And Addiction Disorders

Chapter 28

Eating Disorders

What Are Eating Disorders?[1]

There is a commonly held view that eating disorders are a lifestyle choice. Eating disorders are actually serious and often fatal illnesses that cause severe disturbances to a person's eating behaviors. Obsessions with food, body weight, and shape may also signal an eating disorder. Common eating disorders include anorexia nervosa, bulimia nervosa, and binge eating disorder.

> Eating disorders are real, treatable medical illnesses. They frequently coexist with other illnesses such as depression, substance abuse, or anxiety disorders. Other symptoms can become life-threatening if a person does not receive treatment, which is reflected by anorexia being associated with the highest mortality rate of any psychiatric disorder.
>
> Eating disorders affect both genders, although rates among women and girls are 2½ times greater than among men and boys. Eating disorders frequently appear during the teen years or young adulthood but also may develop during childhood or later in life.
>
> (Source: "Eating Disorders: About More Than Food," National Institute of Mental Health (NIMH).)

This chapter includes text excerpted from documents published by two public domain sources. Text under headings marked 1 is excerpted from "Eating Disorders," National Institute of Mental Health (NIMH), February 2016; Text under heading marked 2 are excerpted from "Eating Disorders: About More Than Food," National Institute of Mental Health (NIMH), 2014.

What Are The Different Types Of Eating Disorders?[2]

The eating disorders anorexia nervosa, bulimia nervosa, and binge eating disorder, and their variants, all feature serious disturbances in eating behavior and weight regulation. They are associated with a wide range of adverse psychological, physical, and social consequences. A person with an eating disorder may start out just eating smaller or larger amounts of food, but at some point, their urge to eat less or more spirals out of control. Severe distress or concern about body weight or shape, or extreme efforts to manage weight or food intake, also may characterize an eating disorder.

Anorexia Nervosa

Many people with anorexia nervosa see themselves as overweight, even when they are clearly underweight. Eating, food, and weight control become obsessions. People with anorexia nervosa typically weigh themselves repeatedly, portion food carefully, and eat very small quantities of only certain foods. Some people with anorexia nervosa also may engage in binge eating followed by extreme dieting, excessive exercise, self-induced vomiting, or misuse of laxatives, diuretics, or enemas.

Symptoms of anorexia nervosa include:

- Extremely low body weight

- Severe food restriction

- Relentless pursuit of thinness and unwillingness to maintain a normal or healthy weight

- Intense fear of gaining weight

- Distorted body image and self-esteem that is heavily influenced by perceptions of body weight and shape, or a denial of the seriousness of low body weight

- Lack of menstruation among girls and women.

Some who have anorexia nervosa recover with treatment after only one episode. Others get well but have relapses. Still others have a more chronic, or long-lasting, form of anorexia nervosa, in which their health declines as they battle the illness.

Other symptoms and medical complications may develop over time, including:

- Thinning of the bones (osteopenia or osteoporosis)

- Brittle hair and nails

- Dry and yellowish skin

- Growth of fine hair all over the body (lanugo)

- Mild anemia, muscle wasting, and weakness

- Severe constipation

- Low blood pressure, or slowed breathing and pulse

- Damage to the structure and function of the heart

- Brain damage

- Multi-organ failure

- Drop in internal body temperature, causing a person to feel cold all the time

- Lethargy, sluggishness, or feeling tired all the time

- Infertility.

Bulimia Nervosa

People with bulimia nervosa have recurrent and frequent episodes of eating unusually large amounts of food and feel a lack of control over these episodes. This binge eating is followed by behavior that compensates for the overeating such as forced vomiting, excessive use of laxatives or diuretics, fasting, excessive exercise, or a combination of these behaviors.

Unlike anorexia nervosa, people with bulimia nervosa usually maintain what is considered a healthy or normal weight, while some are slightly overweight. But like people with anorexia nervosa, they often fear gaining weight, want desperately to lose weight, and are intensely unhappy with their body size and shape. Usually, bulimic behavior is done secretly because it is often accompanied by feelings of disgust or shame. The binge eating and purging cycle can happen anywhere from several times a week to many times a day.

Other symptoms include:

- Chronically inflamed and sore throat

- Swollen salivary glands in the neck and jaw area

- Worn tooth enamel, and increasingly sensitive and decaying teeth as a result of exposure to stomach acid

- Acid reflux disorder and other gastrointestinal problems

- Intestinal distress and irritation from laxative abuse

- Severe dehydration from purging of fluids

- Electrolyte imbalance—too low or too high levels of sodium, calcium, potassium, and other minerals that can lead to a heart attack or stroke.

Binge Eating Disorder

People with binge eating disorder lose control over their eating. Unlike bulimia nervosa, periods of binge eating are not followed by compensatory behaviors like purging, excessive exercise, or fasting. As a result, people with binge eating disorder often are overweight or obese. People with binge eating disorder who are obese are at higher risk for developing cardiovascular disease and high blood pressure. They also experience guilt, shame, and distress about their binge eating, which can lead to more binge eating.

Risk Factors Of Eating Disorders[1]

Eating disorders frequently appear during the teen years or young adulthood but may also develop during childhood or later in life. These disorders affect both genders, although rates among women are greater than among men. Like women who have eating disorders, men also have a distorted sense of body image. For example, men may have muscle dysmorphia, a type of disorder marked by an extreme concern with becoming more muscular.

Researchers are finding that eating disorders are caused by a complex interaction of genetic, biological, behavioral, psychological, and social factors. Researchers are using the latest technology and science to better understand eating disorders.

One approach involves the study of human genes. Eating disorders run in families. Researchers are working to identify deoxyribonucleic acid (DNA) variations that are linked to the increased risk of developing eating disorders.

Brain imaging studies are also providing a better understanding of eating disorders. For example, researchers have found differences in patterns of brain activity in women with eating disorders in comparison with healthy women. This kind of research can help guide the development of new means of diagnosis and treatment of eating disorders.

Types Of Treatments And Therapies[1]

Adequate nutrition, reducing excessive exercise, and stopping purging behaviors are the foundations of treatment. Treatment plans are tailored to individual needs and may include one or more of the following:

- Individual, group, and/or family psychotherapy

- Medical care and monitoring

- Nutritional counseling

- Medications

Psychotherapies

Psychotherapies such as a family-based therapy called the Maudsley approach, where parents of adolescents with anorexia nervosa assume responsibility for feeding their child, appear to be very effective in helping people gain weight and improve eating habits and moods.

To reduce or eliminate binge eating and purging behaviors, people may undergo cognitive behavioral therapy (CBT), which is another type of psychotherapy that helps a person learn how to identify distorted or unhelpful thinking patterns and recognize and change inaccurate beliefs.

Medications

Evidence also suggests that medications such as antidepressants, antipsychotics, or mood stabilizers approved by the U.S. Food and Drug Administration (FDA) may also be helpful for treating eating disorders and other cooccurring illnesses such as anxiety or depression. Check the FDA's Website (www.fda.gov), for the latest information on warnings, patient medication guides, or newly approved medications.

Chapter 29

Anorexia Nervosa

Anorexia nervosa, often called anorexia, is a type of eating disorder. People with anorexia eat so little that they have unhealthy weight loss and become dangerously thin. They may think they are overweight or fat even when they are underweight or thin. Anorexia affects more girls and women than boys and men. Anorexia is a serious health problem that can increase the risk of early death. But people with anorexia can get better with treatment.

What Is Anorexia?

Anorexia nervosa, often called anorexia, is a type of eating disorder. Eating disorders are mental health problems that cause extreme and dangerous eating behaviors. These extreme eating behaviors cause other serious health problems and sometimes death. Some eating disorders also involve extreme exercise.

Women with anorexia severely limit the amount of food they eat to prevent weight gain. People with anorexia usually have an intense fear of gaining weight and may think they are fat even when they are thin. Women with anorexia may also exercise too much so that they do not gain weight. Over time, eating so little food leads to serious health problems and sometimes death.

What Is The Difference Between Anorexia And Other Eating Disorders?

Women with eating disorders, such as anorexia, bulimia, and binge eating disorder, have a mental health condition that affects how they eat, and sometimes how they exercise. These

About This Chapter: This chapter includes text excerpted from "Anorexia Nervosa," Office on Women's Health (OWH), U.S. Department of Health and Human Services (HHS), June 12, 2017.

eating disorders threaten their health. Unlike women with bulimia and binge eating disorder, girls and women with anorexia do not eat enough to sustain basic bodily functions. Women with bulimia and binge eating disorder usually binge, or eat too much while feeling out of control. It is possible to have more than one eating disorder in your lifetime. Regardless of what type of eating disorder you may have, you can get better with treatment.

Who Is At Risk For Anorexia?

Anorexia is more common among girls and women than boys and men. Anorexia is also more common among girls and younger women than older women. On average, girls develop anorexia at 16 or 17. Teen girls between 13 and 19 and young women in their early 20s are most at risk. But eating disorders are happening more often in older women. In a study, 13% of American women over 50 had signs of an eating disorder.

What Are The Symptoms Of Anorexia?

Anorexia causes physical and psychological changes. A girl or woman with anorexia often looks very thin and may not act like herself.

Some other symptoms of anorexia include:

- Sadness

- Moodiness

- Confused or slow thinking

- Poor memory or judgment

- Thin, brittle hair and nails

- Feeling cold all the time because of a drop in internal body temperature

- Feeling faint, dizzy, or weak

- Feeling tired or sluggish

- Irregular periods or never getting a period

- Dry, blotchy, or yellow skin

- Growth of fine hair all over the body (called lanugo)

- Severe constipation or bloating

- Weak muscles or swollen joints

Girls or women with anorexia may also have behavior changes such as:

- Talking about weight or food all the time

- Not eating or eating very little

- Refusing to eat in front of others

- Not wanting to go out with friends

- Making herself throw up

- Taking laxatives or diet pills

- Exercising a lot

People with anorexia may also have other health problems, including depression, anxiety, or substance abuse.

What Causes Anorexia?

Researchers are not sure exactly what causes anorexia and other eating disorders. Researchers think that eating disorders might happen because of a combination of a person's biology and life events. This combination includes having specific genes, a person's biology, body image and self-esteem, social experiences, family health history, and sometimes other mental health illnesses. Researchers are also studying unusual activity in the brain, such as changing levels of serotonin or other chemicals, to see how it may affect eating.

> Anorexia usually begins during the teen years or young adulthood. It is more common in females, but may also be seen in males. The disorder is seen mainly in white women who are high academic achievers and who have a goal-oriented family or personality.
>
> (Source: "Anorexia Nervosa," MentalHealth.gov, U.S. Department of Health and Human Services (HHS).)

How Is Anorexia Diagnosed?

Your doctor or nurse will ask you questions about your symptoms and medical history. It may be difficult to talk to a doctor or nurse about secret eating or exercise behaviors. But doctors and nurses want to help you be healthy. Being honest about your eating and exercise behaviors with a doctor or nurse is a good way to ask for help. Your doctor will do a physical exam and other tests, such as blood tests and a urine test, to rule out other health problems that may cause severe weight loss. Your doctor may also do other tests, such as kidney function tests, bone density tests, or an electrocardiogram (ECG or EKG), to see if or how severe weight loss has affected your health.

How Is Anorexia Treated?

Your doctor may refer you to a team of doctors, nutritionists, and therapists who will work to help you get better. If you live with family members they may be invited to participate in some of your treatment.

Treatment plans may include one or more of the following:

- **Nutrition therapy.** Doctors, nurses, and counselors will help you eat healthy to reach and maintain a healthy weight. Some girls or women may need to be hospitalized or participate in a residential treatment program (live temporarily at a medical facility) to make sure they eat enough to recover. Hospitalization may also be required to monitor any heart problems in people with anorexia. Reaching a healthy weight is a key part of the recovery process so that your body's biology, including thoughts and feelings in your brain, work correctly.

- **Psychotherapy.** Sometimes called "talk therapy," psychotherapy is counseling to help you change any harmful thoughts or behaviors. This therapy may focus on the importance of talking about your feelings and how they affect what you do. You may work one-on-one with a therapist or in a group with others who have anorexia. For girls with anorexia, counseling may involve the whole family.

- **Support groups** can be helpful for some people with anorexia when added to other treatment. In support groups, girls or women and sometimes their families meet and share their stories.

- **Medicine.** Studies suggest that medicines like antidepressants can help some girls and women with anorexia by improving the depression and anxiety symptoms that often go along with anorexia.

Chapter 30

Bulimia Nervosa

Bulimia nervosa, often called bulimia, is a type of eating disorder. People with bulimia eat large amounts of food at one time, then try to get rid of the food or weight gain by throwing up, taking laxatives, fasting (not eating anything), or exercising a lot more than normal. Bulimia affects more girls and women than boys and men. Bulimia is a serious health problem, but people with bulimia can get better with treatment.

> Bulimia nervosa is characterized by recurrent and frequent episodes of eating unusually large amounts of food (e.g., binge-eating), and feeling a lack of control over the eating. This binge-eating is followed by a type of behavior that compensates for the binge, such as purging (e.g., vomiting, excessive use of laxatives or diuretics), fasting and/or excessive exercise. Unlike anorexia nervosa, people with bulimia can fall within the normal range for their weight. But like people with anorexia, they often fear gaining weight, want desperately to lose weight, and are intensely unhappy with their body size and shape.
>
> *(Source: "Eating Disorders Among Adults—Bulimia Nervosa," National Institute of Mental Health (NIMH).)*

What Is Bulimia?

Bulimia nervosa, often called bulimia, is a type of eating disorder. Eating disorders are mental health problems that cause extreme and dangerous eating behaviors. These extreme eating behaviors cause other serious health problems and sometimes death. Some eating disorders

About This Chapter: This chapter includes text excerpted from "Bulimia Nervosa," Office on Women's Health (OWH), U.S. Department of Health and Human Services (HHS), June 26, 2016.

also involve extreme exercise. Women with bulimia eat a lot of food in a short amount of time and feel a lack of control over eating during this time (called binging). People with bulimia then try to prevent weight gain by getting rid of the food (called purging).

Purging may be done by:

- Making yourself throw up

- Taking laxatives. Laxatives can include pills or liquids that speed up the movement of food through your body and lead to bowel movements.

What Is The Difference Between Bulimia And Other Eating Disorders?

Women with eating disorders, such as bulimia, anorexia, and binge eating disorder, have a mental health condition that affects how they eat, and sometimes how they exercise. These eating disorders threaten their health. Unlike women with anorexia, women with bulimia often have a normal weight. Unlike women with binge eating disorder, women with bulimia purge, or try to get rid of the food or weight after binging. Binging and purging are usually done in private. This can make it difficult to tell if a loved one has bulimia or another eating disorder. It is possible to have more than one eating disorder in your lifetime. Regardless of what type of eating disorder you may have, you can get better with treatment.

Who Is At Risk For Bulimia?

Bulimia affects more women than men. It affects up to 2 percent of women and happens to women of all races and ethnicities. Bulimia affects more girls and younger women than older women. On average, women develop bulimia at 18 or 19. Teen girls between 15 and 19 and young women in their early 20s are most at risk. But eating disorders are happening more often in older women. In one recent study, 13 percent of American women over 50 had signs of an eating disorder.

What Are The Symptoms Of Bulimia?

Someone with bulimia may be thin, overweight, or have a normal weight. It can be difficult to tell based on a person's weight whether someone has bulimia. This is because binging and purging is most often done in private. However, family or friends may see empty food wrappers in unexpected places or vomit in the home.

Over time, some symptoms of bulimia may include:

- Swollen cheeks or jaw area

- Calluses or scrapes on the knuckles (if using fingers to induce vomiting)

- Teeth that look clear instead of white and are increasingly sensitive and decaying

- Broken blood vessels in the eyes

- Acid reflux, constipation, and other gastrointestinal problems

- Severe dehydration

Girls or women with bulimia may also have behavior changes such as:

- Often going to the bathroom right after eating (to throw up)

- Exercising a lot, even in bad weather or when hurt or tired

- Acting moody or sad, hating the way she looks, or feeling hopeless

- Having problems expressing anger

- Not wanting to go out with friends or do activities she once enjoyed

People with bulimia often have other mental health problems, including depression, anxiety, or substance abuse.

What Causes Bulimia?

Researchers are not sure exactly what causes bulimia and other eating disorders. Researchers think that eating disorders might happen because of a combination of a person's biology and life events. This combination includes having specific genes, a person's biology, body image and self-esteem, social experiences, family health history, and sometimes other mental health illnesses. Researchers are also studying unusual activity in the brain, such as changing levels of serotonin or other chemicals, to see how it may affect eating.

How Is Bulimia Diagnosed?

Your doctor or nurse will ask you questions about your symptoms and medical history. It may be difficult to talk to a doctor or nurse about secret eating, purging, or exercise behaviors. But doctors and nurses want to help you get better. Being honest about your eating behaviors with a doctor or nurse is a good way to ask for help.

Your doctor may do blood or urine tests to rule out other possible causes of your symptoms. Your doctor may also do other tests to see whether you have any other health problems caused by bulimia. These tests may include kidney function tests or an electrocardiogram (ECG or EKG) to see if or how repeated binging and purging has affected your health.

How Is Bulimia Treated?

Your doctor may refer you to a team of doctors, nutritionists, and therapists who will work to help you get better. Treatment plans may include one or more of the following:

- **Nutrition therapy.** People who purge (make themselves throw up or take laxatives) regularly should be treated by a doctor. Purging can cause life-threatening electrolyte imbalances. Some people with bulimia may need to be hospitalized if they have serious heart or kidney problems.

- **Psychotherapy.** Sometimes called "talk therapy," psychotherapy is counseling to help you change harmful thoughts or behaviors. This type of therapy may focus on the importance of talking about your feelings and how they affect what you do. For example, you might talk about how stress triggers a binge. You may work one-on-one with a therapist or in a group with others who have bulimia.

- **Nutritional counseling.** A registered dietitian or counselor can help you eat in a healthier way than binging and purging.

- **Support groups** can be helpful for some people with bulimia when added to other treatment. In support groups, girls or women and sometimes their families meet and share their stories.

- **Medicine.** Fluoxetine (Prozac) is the only medicine approved by the U.S. Food and Drug Administration (FDA) for treating bulimia, but only in adults. It may help reduce binging and purging and improve your thoughts about eating. Some antidepressants may help girls and women with bulimia who also have depression or anxiety.

Chapter 31

Binge Eating Disorder

Binge eating disorder is the most common type of eating disorder in the United States. People with binge eating disorder often feel out of control and eat a large amount of food at one time (called a binge). Unlike other eating disorders, people who have binge eating disorder do not throw up the food or exercise too much. Binge eating disorder is a serious health problem, but people with binge eating disorder can get better with treatment.

What Is Binge Eating Disorder?

Binge eating disorder is a type of eating disorder. Eating disorders are mental health problems that cause extreme and dangerous eating behaviors. These extreme eating behaviors cause other serious health problems and sometimes death. Some eating disorders also involve extreme exercise. According to the American Psychiatric Association (APA), women with binge eating disorder feel out of control and eat too much (binge), at least once a week for at least three months. During binges, women with binge eating disorder usually eat faster than normal, eat until they are uncomfortable, eat when they are not physically hungry, and feel embarrassed, disgusted, or depressed because of the binges. Women with this type of eating disorder may be overweight or obese.

What Is The Difference Between Binge Eating Disorder And Other Eating Disorders?

Women with eating disorders, such as binge eating disorder, bulimia, and anorexia, have a mental health condition that affects how they eat, and sometimes how they exercise. These

About This Chapter: This chapter includes text excerpted from "Binge Eating Disorder," Office on Women's Health (OWH), U.S. Department of Health and Human Services (HHS), June 26, 2016.

eating disorders threaten their health. Unlike people with anorexia or bulimia, people with binge eating disorder do not throw up their food, exercise a lot, or starve themselves. People with binge eating disorder are often overweight or obese. But not all people with binge eating disorder are overweight, and being overweight does not always mean you have binge eating disorder. It is possible to have more than one eating disorder in your lifetime. Regardless of what type of eating disorder you may have, you can get better with treatment.

Who Is At Risk For Binge Eating Disorder?

Binge eating disorder affects more than 3 percent of women in the United States. More than half of people with binge eating disorder are women. Binge eating disorder affects women of all races and ethnicities. It is the most common eating disorder among Hispanic, Asian-American, and African-American women.

Some women may be more at risk for binge eating disorder.

- Women and girls who diet often are 12 times more likely to binge eat than women and girls who do not diet.

- Binge eating disorder affects more young and middle-aged women than older women. On average, women develop binge eating disorder in their early to mid-20s. But eating disorders are happening more often in older women. In one study, 13 percent of American women over 50 had signs of an eating disorder.

What Are The Symptoms Of Binge Eating Disorder?

It can be difficult to tell whether someone has binge eating disorder. Many women with binge eating disorder hide their behavior because they are embarrassed. You may have binge eating disorder if, for at least once a week over the past three months, you have binged. Binge eating disorder means you have at least three of these symptoms while binging:

- Eating faster than normal
- Eating until uncomfortably full
- Eating large amounts of food when not hungry
- Eating alone because of embarrassment
- Feeling disgusted, depressed, or guilty afterward

People with binge eating disorder may also have other mental health problems, such as depression, anxiety, or substance abuse.

What Causes Binge Eating Disorder?

Researchers are not sure exactly what causes binge eating disorder and other eating disorders. Researchers think that eating disorders might happen because of a combination of a person's biology and life events. This combination includes having specific genes, a person's biology, body image and self-esteem, social experiences, family health history, and sometimes other mental health illnesses. Studies suggest that people with binge eating disorder may use overeating as a way to deal with anger, sadness, boredom, anxiety, or stress. Researchers are studying how changing levels of brain chemicals may affect eating habits. Neuroimaging, or pictures of the brain, may lead to a better understanding of binge eating disorder.

How Is Binge Eating Disorder Diagnosed?

Your doctor or nurse will ask you questions about your symptoms and medical history. It may be difficult to talk to a doctor or nurse about secret eating behaviors. But doctors and nurses want to help you be healthy. Being honest about your eating behaviors with a doctor or nurse is a good way to ask for help. Your doctor may also do blood, urine, or other tests for other health problems, such as heart problems or gallbladder disease, that can be caused by binge eating disorder.

Talk to your doctor if you think you have binge eating disorder. Ask him or her to refer you to a mental health professioinal in your area. A specialist, such as a psychiatrist, psychologist or other mental health professional, may be able to help you choose the best treatment for you.

Treatment may include therapy to help you change your eating habits, as well as thoughts and feelings that may lead to binge eating and other psychological symptoms. Types of therapy that have been shown to help people with binge eating disorder are called psychotherapies and include cognitive behavioral therapy, interpersonal psychotherapy, and dialectical behavior therapy. Your psychiatrist or other healthcare provider may also prescribe medication to help you with your binge eating, or to treat other medical or mental health problems.

(Source: "Diagnosis And Treatment Of Binge Eating Disorder," National Institute of Diabetes and Digestive and Kidney Diseases (NIDDK).)

How Is Binge Eating Disorder Treated?

Your doctor may refer you to a team of doctors, nutritionists, and therapists who will work to help you get better. Treatment plans may include one or more of the following:

- **Psychotherapy.** Sometimes called "talk therapy," psychotherapy is counseling to help you change any harmful thoughts or behaviors. This therapy may focus on the importance of talking about your feelings and how they affect what you do. For example, you might talk about how stress triggers a binge. You may work one-on-one with a therapist or in a group with others who have binge eating disorder.

- **Nutritional counseling.** A registered dietitian can help you eat in a healthier way.

- **Medicine,** such as appetite suppressants or antidepressants prescribed by a doctor. Antidepressants may help some girls and women with binge eating disorder who also have anxiety or depression.

Most girls and women do get better with treatment and are able to eat in healthy ways again. Some may get better after the first treatment. Others get well but may relapse and need treatment again.

Chapter 32

Body Dysmorphic Disorder

Do you like what you see when you look in the mirror? If your answer is "No," you're not alone. For many of us, there's a growing gap between how our bodies look and how we'd like them to look.

Americans have generally gotten wider and flabbier over the past few decades, as obesity rates continue to climb. But at the same time, the media bombard us with images of people who seem impossibly thin or muscular. The gap between reality and expectations can leave many people feeling inadequate.

It's normal to look in the mirror occasionally and wish for a firmer body or more glamorous hair. But some people find they can't stop thinking about body flaws they believe they have. They may avoid going out with friends or even stop going to work because they feel ashamed of their skin, hair, weight or other features.

"They say they look ugly, flawed or deformed, but in reality they look fine," says Dr. Katharine A. Phillips, a psychiatrist at Brown University. "The physical flaws they perceive are things we can't see at all, or they're really quite minimal."

Having a negative body image like this isn't just an attitude problem. It can take a toll on your mental and physical health. If excessive thoughts about your body cause great distress or

About This Chapter: Text in this chapter begins with experts from "How You See Yourself—When Your Body Image Doesn't Measure Up," *NIH News in Health*, National Institutes of Health (NIH), July 2009. Reviewed July 2017; Text under the heading "What Is Body Dysmorphic Disorder (BDD)?" is excerpted from "Cognitive-Behavioral Therapy And Supportive Psychotherapy For Body Dysmorphic Disorder," ClinicalTrials.gov, National Institutes of Health (NIH), March 15, 2016; Text beginning with the heading "Symptoms Of BDD" is excerpted from "Body Image—Cosmetic Surgery," Office on Women's Health (OWH), U.S. Department of Health and Human Services (HHS), September 22, 2009. Reviewed July 2017.

interfere with your daily life, you may have a body image disorder, also known as body dysmorphic disorder (BDD).

What Is Body Dysmorphic Disorder (BDD)?

Body dysmorphic disorder (BDD) is a severe, often chronic, and common disorder consisting of distressing or impairing preoccupation with perceived defects in one's physical appearance. Individuals with BDD have very poor psychosocial functioning and high rates of hospitalization and suicidality. Because BDD differs in important ways from other disorders, psychotherapies for other disorders are not adequate for BDD. Despite BDD's severity, there is no adequately tested psychosocial treatment (psychotherapy) of any type for this disorder.

Symptoms Of BDD

- Being preoccupied with minor or imaginary physical flaws, usually of the skin, hair, and nose, such as acne, scarring, facial lines, marks, pale skin, thinning hair, excessive body hair, large nose, or crooked nose.

- Having a lot of anxiety and stress about the perceived flaw and spending a lot of time focusing on it, such as frequently picking at skin, excessively checking appearance in a mirror, hiding the imperfection, comparing appearance with others, excessively grooming, seeking reassurance from others about how they look, and getting cosmetic surgery.

> Getting cosmetic surgery can make BDD worse. They are often not happy with the outcome of the surgery. If they are, they may start to focus attention on another body area and become preoccupied trying to fix the new "defect." In this case, some patients with BDD become angry at the surgeon for making their appearance worse and may even become violent towards the surgeon.

Treatment For BDD

- **Medications.** Serotonin reuptake inhibitors or SSRIs are antidepressants that decrease the obsessive and compulsive behaviors.

- **Cognitive behavioral therapy.** This is a type of therapy with several steps:

  1. The therapist asks the patient to enter social situations without covering up her "defect."

2. The therapist helps the patient stop doing the compulsive behaviors to check the defect or cover it up. This may include removing mirrors, covering skin areas that the patient picks, or not using make-up.

3. The therapist helps the patient change their false beliefs about their appearance.

Chapter 33

Compulsive Exercise Disorder

What Is Compulsive Exercise?

Compulsive exercise (also known as anorexia athletica) is a type of addiction in which a person feels that they must work out frequently, often several times a day, and feels anxious and guilty if they don't work out enough. For those struggling with a compulsive exercise disorder, working out is not a choice. Exercise becomes an obligation, one that takes over the person's life to an extreme degree. Working out becomes the most important priority, often at the expense of other activities. A person with compulsive exercise disorder will strive to work out even with an injury or illness that would normally prevent physical exertion. For this reason, compulsive exercise often creates severe physical and psychological problems.

Research has shown that the majority of people with compulsive exercise disorder are female. Many people exercise compulsively in order to feel more in control of their lives, and they define their self-worth through athletic achievements. Some use exercise as a way to try to handle difficult emotions or depression, believing that physical exhaustion will eliminate negative feelings. Others develop compulsive exercise disorder through participation in competitive sports. External and internal pressure to succeed or excel in sports can drive an athlete to push workouts too far, too frequently. In these cases, exercise compulsion is driven by the belief that additional workouts will provide the edge needed to win.

Compulsive exercise (also known as anorexia athletica) is a type of addiction in which a person feels that they must work out frequently, often several times a day, and feels anxious and guilty if they don't work out enough. For those struggling with a compulsive exercise disorder, working out is not a choice. Exercise becomes an obligation, one that takes over the person's life to an extreme degree. Working out becomes the most important priority, often at the expense of other activities. A person with compulsive exercise disorder will strive to work out even with an injury or illness that would normally prevent physical exertion. For this reason, compulsive exercise often creates severe physical and psychological problems.

Maintaining Body Weight

Try to maintain your body weight by balancing what you eat with physical activity. If you are sedentary, try to become more active. If you are already very active, try to continue the same level of activity as you age. More physical activity is better than less, and any is better than none. If your weight is not in the healthy range, try to reduce health risks through better eating and exercise habits. Take steps to keep your weight within the healthy range (neither too high nor too low). Have children's heights and weights checked regularly by a health professional.

(Source: "Balance The Food You Eat With Physical Activity—Maintain Or Improve Your Weight," U.S. Department of Health and Human Services (HHS).)

If You Need To Lose Weight

You do not need to lose weight if your weight is already within the healthy range in the figure, if you have gained less than 10 pounds since you reached your adult height, and if you are otherwise healthy. If you are overweight and have excess abdominal fat, a weight-related medical problem, or a family history of such problems, you need to lose weight. Healthy diets and exercise can help people maintain a healthy weight, and may also help them lose weight. It is important to recognize that overweight is a chronic condition which can only be controlled with long-term changes. To reduce caloric intake, eat less fat and control portion sizes. If you are not physically active, spend less time in sedentary activities such as watching television, and be more active throughout the day. As people lose weight, the body becomes more efficient at using energy and the rate of weight loss may decrease. Increased physical activity will help you to continue losing weight and to avoid gaining it back.

(Source: "Balance The Food You Eat With Physical Activity—Maintain Or Improve Your Weight," U.S. Department of Health and Human Services (HHS).)

Health Effects Of Compulsive Exercise Disorder

Compulsive exercise is dangerous and can result in serious physical and psychological harm.

Stress fractures can develop in weight-bearing areas of the body (such as feet and lower legs) as a result of repetitive, high-impact, weight-bearing activities such as running or jumping.

Stress fractures produce pain during exercise and can develop into more serious bone breaks if not allowed to heal properly.

Consider This

People who exercise compulsively often believe they are improving their health, but the negative effects of too much exercise can result in serious complications.

Damage to muscle and connective tissue is one common side effect of compulsive exercise. Fitness experts advocate for periods of rest between workouts to allow the body to heal from minor injuries and muscle strains. Long-term damage can result from insufficient rest time, including loss of muscle mass, particularly for those who also struggle with eating disorders. A malnourished body begins to break down muscle tissue for fuel when calories are not available to burn.

Low heart rate (bradycardia) is a condition that develops from metabolic disruptions due to over-exercising. The body's normal response to rapid weight loss is to slow the metabolism in an effort to burn as few calories as possible. Low heart rate typically results in low body temperature and decreased resting heart rate. Low heart rate can easily be mistaken as a positive result of exercise, but in cases of exercise compulsion, low heart rate can produce serious arrhythmias (irregular heart function) and even sudden death.

Osteoporosis results in bone loss which increases the risk of stress fractures. This is a particularly dangerous risk for those suffering from both compulsive exercise and eating disorders, due to malnutrition from a poor diet.

Amenorrhea is the loss of normal menstruation that often develops during rapid and severe weight loss. Amenorrhea can result in loss of bone density and other serious problems including reproductive issues.

Exercising to the point of exhaustion on a frequent basis overloads the body with adrenaline and cortisol hormones, which in turn compromise the body's natural immune system. This increases the likelihood of illness, fatigue, insomnia or other sleep-related problems, irritability, short attention span, and mood swings.

Did You Know?

Compulsive exercise can lead to other dangerous conditions such as bulimia, anorexia, obsessive-compulsive disorder, negative thinking, low self-esteem, and social isolation.

Signs And Symptoms Of Compulsive Exercise Disorder

Some of the warning signs of a compulsive exercise disorder include:

- Feeling guilty, anxious, or irritable about missing workouts

- Pushing yourself to exercise even when injured or ill

- Persistent exhaustion and fatigue

- Chronic insomnia or disrupted sleep

- Slower than normal heart rate

- Inability to rest or even to sit still

- Giving up social time with friends in order to work out

- Obsessive focus on the number of calories eaten and burned

- Constantly thinking about working out

- Working out even in bad weather

- Low body weight, being underweight for your height

- Feeling obligated to exercise

- Lack of enjoyment of physical activity

- Making up for eating by exercising more

- Lack of satisfaction from personal achievements, always feeling there is more to do

Treatment Of Compulsive Exercise Disorder

Treatment and recovery from compulsive exercise disorder can take months to years, depending on the individual person and situation. Some common treatment approaches include psychotherapy and medication to help manage compulsive disorders. Cognitive behavioral therapy can help to identify and correct negative thoughts and attitudes. Therapy can also help provide healthy strategies to address negative emotions, stress, low self-esteem and negative body image. Family therapy can be useful when external pressures to excel may have inadvertently caused a compulsive exercise disorder. Family members may not be aware of overly high expectations and the resulting stress that is placed on a young person. This can be particularly critical for athletes who participate in sports that emphasize being thin, such as ice skating, gymnastics, and dancing. Participating in these sports can create an unhealthy focus on body weight.

References

1. "Compulsive Exercise," KidsHealth, October 2013.

2. "Compulsive Exercise: Are You Overdoing It?" WebMD, February 26, 2016.

3. "Exercise Compulsion and Its Dangers," Eating Disorder Hope, October 5, 2012.

Chapter 34

Impulse Control Disorders

Impulse control disorders (ICDs) are a group of disorders in which a person is unable to resist the impulse to do something negative even though it has harmful consequences. Research indicated that of those American diagnosed with a mental health disorder, 10 percent of them suffer from impulse control disorder (ICD).

People with ICD experience a regular, overwhelming desire to engage in a negative behavior and progressive lack of control. Performing the negative behavior will provide them a sense of relief or pleasure.

Impulse control disorders are seen more in males than in females and they generally coexist with an underlying mental health disorder like substance abuse. It can be challenging to identify individuals with ICD as they may not seek help.

The medical community classifies the following disorders under impulse control disorders:

- **Intermittent explosive disorder (IED)**—This disorder is characterized by uncontrolled fits of extreme anger and violence. People with this disorder usually allow their negative behavior to grow out of control, and, in the long run, their actions result in legal or financial issues, disrupt interpersonal relationships, and potentially result in problems at work or school.

- **Kleptomania**—Kleptomania is characterized by an irresistible compulsion to steal. Those who suffer from the disorder do not steal because they desire an object or seek financial gain. Their only motivation is to satisfy their desire to steal. Following an episode the person will feel intense guilt and shame.

"Impulse Control Disorders," © 2017 Omnigraphics. Reviewed July 2017.

- **Pyromania**—Pyromaniacs have irresistible urges to set fires. Again, the person does this out of mental compulsion with no other intention.

- **Conduct disorder**—A disorder that involves an individual displaying repetitive and persistent behaviors that violate social norms and the rights of others.

Other disorders include:

- **Exhibitionism**—Compulsive need to expose one's genitals to an unsuspecting stranger.

- **Pathological gambling**—Uncontrollable addiction to gambling.

- **Trichotillomania**—Individuals with this disorder compulsively twist and pull their hair, often resulting in bald spots.

What Are The Causes Of Impulse Control Disorders?

The exact cause of impulse control disorder is, however, medical professionals generally agree that a combination of various factors, including biological, environmental, psychological, and even cultural or societal factors, may play a role in causing this disorder.

Recent research has also indicated that these disorders may be caused by a neurotransmitter imbalance in the brain as well as hormonal imbalances, such as elevated testosterone levels, that can result in aggressive behaviors.

Other risk factors, including stressful living conditions, childhood trauma or neglect, and mitigating environmental factors, may also influence the disorder's onset. Medical disorders such as seizures may cause trauma to the brain resulting in impulse control disorder.

Preexisting mental health disorders such as substance abuse can alter the brain's chemistry and thereby increase the risk of impulse control disorders.

How Are Impulse Control Disorders Treated?

Since a combination of factors cause impulse control disorders, treatment also typically involves a combination of methods and usually involves medication, psychotherapy, and behavioral modification therapy.

- Cognitive therapy will encourage the individual to identify negative behavioral patterns and the negative consequences associated with those behaviors.

- Behavioral modification therapy will teach new coping mechanisms and techniques on how to avoid situations leading to impulsive behaviors. Cognitive behavioral therapy has been widely used and it is found to be an effective one.

- Exposure therapy places the individual in the situations leading to impulsive behaviors while working with him or her to exercise self-control. This helps the person to gradually build tolerance to the situation gradually and respond appropriately.

- Other complimentary methods, such as mindfulness techniques, yoga or meditation, hypnotism, and herbal remedies, can also be beneficial in helping people learn how to improve willpower and control emotions when faced with stressors.

- Although no drugs are specially approved in the treatment of impulse control disorder, some medications have proven effective in some cases. Selective serotonin reuptake inhibitors (SSRIs) are antidepressant medications that have shown effectiveness in treating impulse control disorders.

Before starting a medication to treat an impulse control disorder, patient should be screened for drug and alcohol addiction. This will help avoid unnecessary complications and ensure safe care for the individual. If an individual is addicted, he or she should undergo a detox program before starting medication for impulse control disorder.

References

1. "Impulse Control Disorder and Abuse," American Addiction Centers, n.d.

2. "The State of Mental Health in America," Mental Health America (MHA), n.d.

3. "Impulse Control Disorders," Disorders.org, n.d.

4. Patricelli, Kathryn. "Impulse Control Disorder," Gulf Bend Center, n.d.

5. "Impulse Control Disorder," East Central Mental Health Center, n.d.

Chapter 35

Adjustment Disorders

What Is Adjustment Disorder?

Adjustment disorder is a stress-related condition in which a person experiences an unusually long-lasting reaction to an unexpected and stressful event. Generally, people get over stressful events in a few months. But people with adjustment disorder continue to have emotional and behavioral responses that lead to anxiety and depression. They experience feelings of sadness, hopelessness, and sometimes physical symptoms significant enough to disrupt relationships and affect work or school life. The disorder is the result of an inability to cope and come to terms with the stressful event. It is mostly seen in children and adolescents but can also occur in adults.

What Causes Adjustment Disorder?

An upsetting or stressful event such as death of a loved one, a failed relationship or divorce, a major disappointment in life, starting a new school, or a financial crisis can trigger adjustment disorder. Whatever the trigger, the event becomes hard for the person to handle. He or she often attributes greater importance to it over a longer period of time than those around them and their reactions are often severe. Children could become anxious, refuse to go to school, become hostile, or get into regular fights.

What Are The Risk Factors For Adjustment Disorder?

No one reacts in the same way to stressful events, and it is hard to predict if someone will develop adjustment disorder. Social skills developed by a person are an important factor that determines if they are particularly vulnerable to this disorder. The disorder is seen across cultures and the exact stressors are often based on cultural influences.

What Are The Symptoms Of Adjustment Disorder?

In adjustment disorder, the reaction to a stressful event is excessive compared to what is normally expected. Symptoms are significant enough to cause problems in social, work, and educational circles. Behavioral patterns vary in children and adults. Children and adolescents exhibit behavioral symptoms such as acting out, while adults exhibit depressive symptoms. The following symptoms are seen in people with adjustment disorder:

- Trouble sleeping

- Anxiety

- Vandalism and fighting in school

- Avoiding school

- Finding it difficult to carry on with daily activities

- Defiance and impulsive actions

- Irritability

- Crying spells

- Feelings of hopelessness

- Becoming withdrawn and staying away from people

- Suicidal ideation

How Is Adjustment Disorder Diagnosed?

The diagnosis of adjustment disorder by a psychiatrist begins with a comprehensive psychological evaluation. This includes development history, life events, behavior and emotions displayed by the person. The doctor uses criteria laid out in the *Diagnostic and Statistical Manual of Mental Disorders*, Fifth Edition (DSM-5) during evaluation. Any major incident in the past that could be a likely stressor and associated symptoms are identified. The psychiatrist also rules out other mental disorders that may be the cause of symptoms.

The DSM-5 lists six types of adjustment disorders:

1. **With depressed mood.** Symptoms include feelings of sadness, hopelessness, feeling tearful, and lacking pleasure in doing things that were previously enjoyable.

2. **With anxiety.** Fear of separation from parents, nervousness, worry, and becoming overwhelmed are seen.

3. **With mixed anxiety and depressed mood.** Symptoms are a combination of anxiety and depression.

4. **With disturbance of conduct.** Behavioral problems present in the form of disruptive actions such as fighting, vandalism, reckless driving, and skipping school are observed.

5. **With mixed disturbance of emotions and conduct.** Symptoms are a combination of depression, anxiety, and behavioral issues.

6. **Unspecified.** Symptoms that don't fit regular definitions, but problems such as difficulty with friends, family, work, and with peers at school can be identified.

Adjustment disorder can be acute or chronic based on how long symptoms last. Acute adjustment disorder lasts for about six months and the outcome is better once the stress-causing factor is resolved. Chronic adjustment disorder lasts beyond six months and causes disruptions in daily functioning.

Because symptoms of adjustment disorder resembles other medical and mental conditions, consulting with a psychiatrist or qualified mental health professional is highly recommended.

How Is Adjustment Disorder Treated?

Adjustment disorder is treated with psychotherapy, medications, or sometimes with both.

Psychotherapy

Psychotherapy or talk therapy is the primary form of treatment recommended for adjustment disorder. In psychotherapy, the patient receives emotional support and therapy focuses on understanding how to cope with negative thoughts and return to normal life and activities. The therapist will take into account various factors such as symptoms, general temperament, and expectations before recommending family therapy, peer group therapy, or cognitive behavior therapy for the patient.

Medications

Mediation is prescribed in cases of depression or anxiety. The regimen might be required only for a few months.

Such medications should be stopped only under a doctor's supervision, since withdrawal symptoms can be severe.

How Can Adjustment Disorder Be Prevented?

Adjustment disorder cannot be prevented, but with professional help it can be identified early on and its effects minimized.

References

1. Mayo Clinic Staff. "Adjustment Disorders," Mayo Clinic, March 10, 2017.

2. "Adjustment Disorders," The Johns Hopkins University, n.d.

3. "Adjustment Disorder Basics," Child Mind Institute, Inc., 2107.

4. Berger, Fred K., MD. "Adjustment Disorders," A.D.A.M., Inc., February 2, 2016.

Chapter 36

Disruptive Behavior Disorders

What Are Disruptive Behavior Disorders (DBDs)?

Disruptive behavior disorders (DBDs) are disorders in which children or teens have trouble controlling their emotions and behavior. Their behavior may be very defiant, and they may strongly conflict with authority figures. Their actions may be aggressive and destructive. All children have mild behavior problems now and then, but DBDs are more severe and continue over time.

DBDs can start when a child is young. Children or teens with a DBD who do not receive treatment often have serious behavior problems at home, at school, or both. They are also more likely to have problems with alcohol or drug use and violent or criminal behavior as they get older. Examples of DBDs include oppositional defiant disorder, conduct disorder, and intermittent explosive disorder.

Oppositional Defiant Disorder

Children or teens with this disorder may have an angry or irritable mood much of the time. They may argue often and refuse to obey parents, caregivers, teachers, or others. They may also want to hurt someone they think has harmed them.

Conduct Disorder

Children or teens with this disorder may act aggressively toward people, animals, or both. They may bully or threaten someone, start physical fights, use weapons, hurt animals, or force

About This Chapter: This chapter includes text excerpted from "Treating Disruptive Behavior Disorders In Children And Teens," Agency for Healthcare Research and Quality (AHRQ), U.S. Department of Health and Human Services (HHS), August 2016.

sexual activity on others. They may also destroy property by fire or other means, lie often, or steal. They may stay out late at night, skip school, or run away from home. They may also lack compassion and not feel guilty about harming others.

Intermittent Explosive Disorder

Children or teens with this disorder may have outbursts of aggressive, violent behavior or shouting. They may have extreme temper tantrums and may start physical fights. They often overreact to situations in extreme ways and do not think about consequences. Outbursts happen with little or no warning. They usually last for 30 minutes or less. After the outburst, the child or teen may feel sorry or embarrassed.

How Common Are DBDs? What Causes Them?

DBDs are one of the most common types of behavioral disorders in children and teens.

- Out of every 100 children in the United States, about 3 of them have a DBD.

- More boys than girls have a DBD.

- DBDs are more common among children aged 12 years and older.

The cause of DBDs is not known. Things that increase the risk for a DBD include:

- Child abuse or neglect

- A traumatic life experience, such as sexual abuse or violence

- A family history of DBDs

Having a child or teen with a DBD can be very stressful for parents, caregivers, and the whole family. But, there are treatments that may help.

How Are DBDs Treated?

To treat your child's or teen's DBD, your healthcare professional may recommend psychosocial treatment (treatment with a trained therapist). If needed, your child's or teen's healthcare professional may also suggest taking a medicine with the psychosocial treatment. Each child or teen responds differently to different treatments. You may need to try several treatments before finding one that is right for your child or teen.

Treatment For Disruptive Behavior Disorders

Starting treatment early is important. Treatment is most effective if it fits the needs of the specific child and family. The first step to treatment is to talk with a healthcare provider. A comprehensive evaluation by a mental health professional may be needed to get the right diagnosis. Some of the signs of behavior problems, such as not following rules in school, could be related to learning problems which may need additional intervention. For younger children, the treatment with the strongest evidence is behavior therapy training for parents, where a therapist helps the parent learn effective ways to strengthen the parent-child relationship and respond to the child's behavior. For school-age children and teens, an often-used effective treatment is a combination of training and therapy that includes the child, the family, and the school.

(Source: "Children's Mental Health—Types Of Disorders," Centers for Disease Control and Prevention (CDC).)

Psychosocial Treatment

Psychosocial treatment can help improve interactions between you and your child or teen. This is done through programs in which parents and their child or teen meet with a trained therapist. It is important for parents and caregivers to be involved in the treatment.

Some programs focus only on parent training. Other programs also work with the child or teen, the whole family together, or with the child's or teen's teachers.

Parent and child training programs are sometimes done in groups. Sessions usually last 1 to 2 hours and are held each week for 8 to 18 weeks. The programs usually charge a fee. Your insurance may cover some of the costs.

Child programs

These programs can help children:

- Feel more positive about themselves and their family

- Strengthen their social, communication, and problem-solving skills

- Better communicate feelings and manage anger

- Practice good behaviors

Teen programs

For teens, a trained therapist may meet with parents and also with the whole family together. The therapist may look for patterns in the way family members interact that could cause tension and problems. The therapist can then help your family learn new ways to communicate to avoid conflict.

The therapist can help you learn how to:

- Be more involved with your teen

- Set clear rules and consequences for breaking the rules

- Improve your leadership, communication, and problem solving skills

- Support your teen

Medicines

Medicines are usually given to children or teens with a DBD only if psychosocial treatment alone does not help enough. Medicines are usually taken together with psychosocial treatment.

Several types of medicines have been used to treat DBDs. These medicines cannot cure DBDs. They are used to reduce symptoms and improve quality of life. The medicines work by changing the way certain chemicals act in the brain.

Medicines work differently in different children or teens. You may have to try several medicines to find one that works for your child or teen.

Chapter 37

Comorbidity: Addiction And Other Mental Disorders

What Is Comorbidity?

The term "comorbidity" describes two or more disorders or illnesses occurring in the same person. They can occur at the same time or one after the other. Comorbidity also implies interactions between the illnesses that can worsen the course of both.

Is Drug Addiction A Mental Illness?

Yes. Addiction changes the brain in fundamental ways, disturbing a person's normal hierarchy of needs and desires and substituting new priorities connected with procuring and using the drug. The resulting compulsive behaviors that weaken the ability to control impulses, despite the negative consequences, are similar to hallmarks of other mental illnesses.

How Common Are Comorbid Drug Addiction And Other Mental Illnesses?

Many people who are addicted to drugs are also diagnosed with other mental disorders and vice versa. For example, compared with the general population, people addicted to drugs are roughly twice as likely to suffer from mood and anxiety disorders, with the reverse also true.

About This Chapter: This chapter includes text excerpted from "DrugFacts—Comorbidity: Addiction And Other Mental Disorders," National Institute on Drug Abuse (NIDA), March 2011. Reviewed July 2017.

Why Do These Disorders Often Cooccur?

Although drug use disorders commonly occur with other mental illnesses, this does not mean that one caused the other, even if one appeared first. In fact, establishing which came first or why can be difficult. However, research suggests the following possibilities for this common cooccurrence:

- **Drug abuse may bring about symptoms of another mental illness.** Increased risk of psychosis in vulnerable marijuana users suggests this possibility.

- **Mental disorders can lead to drug abuse**, possibly as a means of "self-medication." Patients suffering from anxiety or depression may rely on alcohol, tobacco, and other drugs to temporarily alleviate their symptoms.

These disorders could also be caused by shared risk factors, such as:

- **Overlapping genetic vulnerabilities.** Predisposing genetic factors may make a person susceptible to both addiction and other mental disorders or to having a greater risk of a second disorder once the first appears.

- **Overlapping environmental triggers.** Stress, trauma (such as physical or sexual abuse), and early exposure to drugs are common environmental factors that can lead to addiction and other mental illnesses.

- **Involvement of similar brain regions.** Brain systems that respond to reward and stress, for example, are affected by drugs of abuse and may show abnormalities in patients with certain mental disorders.

- **Drug use disorders and other mental illnesses are developmental disorders.** That means they often begin in the teen years or even younger—periods when the brain experiences dramatic developmental changes. Early exposure to drugs of abuse may change the brain in ways that increase the risk for mental disorders. Also, early symptoms of a mental disorder may indicate an increased risk for later drug use.

How Are These Comorbid Conditions Diagnosed And Treated?

The high rate of comorbidity between drug use disorders and other mental illnesses calls for a comprehensive approach that identifies and evaluates both. Accordingly, anyone seeking help for either drug abuse/addiction or another mental disorder should be checked for both and treated accordingly.

Several behavioral therapies have shown promise for treating comorbid conditions. These approaches can be tailored to patients according to age, specific drug abused, and other factors. Some therapies have proven more effective for adolescents, while others have shown greater effectiveness for adults; some are designed for families and groups, others for individuals.

Effective medications exist for treating opioid, alcohol, and nicotine addiction and for alleviating the symptoms of many other mental disorders, yet most have not been well studied in comorbid populations. Some medications may benefit multiple problems. For example, evidence suggests that bupropion (trade names: Wellbutrin, Zyban), approved for treating depression and nicotine dependence, might also help reduce craving and use of the drug methamphetamine. More research is needed, however, to better understand how these medications work, particularly when combined in patients with comorbidities.

How Should Comorbid Conditions Be Treated?

A fundamental principle emerging from scientific research is the need to treat comorbid conditions concurrently—which can be a difficult proposition. Patients who have both a drug use disorder and another mental illness often exhibit symptoms that are more persistent, severe, and resistant to treatment compared with patients who have either disorder alone. Nevertheless, steady progress is being made through research on new and existing treatment options for comorbidity and through health services research on implementation of appropriate screening and treatment within a variety of settings, including criminal justice systems.

(Source: "Comorbidity: Addiction And Other Mental Illnesses," National Institute on Drug Abuse (NIDA).)

Part Five
Other Situations And Disorders With Mental Health Consequences

Chapter 38

Puberty And Its Relationship To Mental Health

Adolescence can be a bewildering time—for both teens and their parents. Yet it can also be thrilling to watch kids grow and change. Learning about teenage development and behaviors can help parents nurture their children's strengths and shepherd them over the rough spots.

Teenagers (15–17 Years Of Age)

This is a time of changes for how teenagers think, feel, and interact with others, and how their bodies grow. Most girls will be physically mature by now, and most will have completed puberty. Boys might still be maturing physically during this time. Your teen might have concerns about her body size, shape, or weight. Eating disorders also can be common, especially among girls. During this time, your teen is developing his unique personality and opinions. Relationships with friends are still important, yet your teen will have other interests as he develops a more clear sense of who he is. This is also an important time to prepare for more independence and responsibility; many teenagers start working, and many will be leaving home soon after high school.

Here is some information on how teens develop:

Emotional/Social Changes

Children in this age group might:

- Have more interest in the opposite sex.
- Go through less conflict with parents.
- Show more independence from parents.

About This Chapter: This chapter includes text excerpted from "Risky Business," *NIH News in Health,* National Institutes of Health (NIH), September 2011. Reviewed July 2017.

- Have a deeper capacity for caring and sharing and for developing more intimate relationships.
- Spend less time with parents and more time with friends.
- Feel a lot of sadness or depression, which can lead to poor grades at school, alcohol or drug use, unsafe sex, and other problems.

Thinking and Learning

Children in this age group might:

- Learn more defined work habits.
- Show more concern about future school and work plans.
- Be better able to give reasons for their own choices, including about what is right or wrong.

(Source: "Child Development—Parenting Tips," Centers for Disease Control and Prevention (CDC).)

Why Does Adolescence Feel So Complicated And Intense?

It all begins with the brain. National Institutes of Health (NIH)-funded scientists have been using advanced imaging tools to take a good look at how the adolescent brain functions. They've found something they didn't expect. Although the 18th birthday means legal adulthood, important regions of the brain are still under construction until about age 25. These still-developing brain areas govern judgment, decision-making, and impulse control.

The adolescent brain can be somewhat like a rider on a racehorse with no reins. "The problem is that the incentive/reward system matures earlier than the cognitive control system," explains Dr. Lisa Freund, a developmental psychologist and neuroscientist at NIH. In other words, the brain's "that's so cool, I want it now" part develops well before the "stop and think twice" part. That's why adolescents are especially susceptible to the immediate rewards of addiction, sexual experience, risky driving and more.

Why Is Adolescence So Risky?

Adolescents have trouble controlling impulses and considering the possible long-term consequences of their actions. What worries parents so much is that kids don't seem to realize how vulnerable they are to the risks they face. Take sex. Among U.S. high school students surveyed in 2009, almost half reported that they had engaged in sexual intercourse at least once, and over 400,000 15- to 19-year-old girls gave birth. Of the 19 million new sexually transmitted diseases (STDs) recorded each year, nearly half are among young people who are 15 to 24 years old. This age group is also the fastest-growing group of people living with human immunodeficiency virus (HIV) in the United States. It's important for parents to take the lead in talking about sex. "Sex is a normal part of life," says Dr. Lynne Haverkos, an NIH pediatrician specializing in health risk behaviors, "but how do you prevent the STDs, pregnancy and negative emotional consequences that can happen in these relationships?

Middle childhood is the time to start talking and listening—then, as they grow, adolescents can develop negotiation skills and learn how to recognize and handle risky situations involving sex. Start communicating early, keep going, don't ever give up."

Talking about sex may feel uncomfortable to some, but parents don't have to go it alone. You can find helpful resources online and in community and school programs. The most effective programs for HIV/STD prevention are taught by trained instructors, are age-appropriate, focus on skill-building and involve parents and health organizations.

You also need to talk to your teen about other behaviors such as drinking alcohol. Alcohol depresses cognitive control and increases the risk for substance abuse and sexual activity. Alcohol and drug use might also lead to situations where teens can be sexually abused.

Why Do Adolescents Need Limits?

Teens may not want limits, but they still need them. Throughout late adolescence and early adulthood, they still need guidance. Setting limits is important because it takes years for kids to master the art of making decisions. Adolescents are similar to preschoolers in that activation in various parts of the brain isn't yet mature and interconnected. "This makes adolescents more emotionally reactive, especially around peers," Freund says.

As the brain's complex architecture develops, teens do begin to learn from experience and adjust their behavior accordingly. They gain the ability to grasp the wider world in more complex and nuanced ways. This helps them develop their sense of right and wrong, as well as objectivity, empathy, and judgment. They may become more motivated by self-esteem and personal achievement. Parents can help by encouraging their teen's strengths. Talking, listening, and channeling an adolescent's ongoing interests can have a powerful positive effect.

When talking with adolescents, "the tone has to be nonjudgmental," says Kapogiannis. "Talk it through, and reassure them that whatever happens, you still love them. As long as you have communication, you're gonna get there."

Freund suggests that parents use technologies—such as texting or mobile phone calls—to stay in contact with their teens. Even if you can't be there physically, they should know that you're available and that you care about them. "You're not hovering, but they need to know you're around," Freund says.

If you have concerns about your teen, and he or she seems unwilling to talk about it, consider making a call to your child's doctor—ideally, an adolescent medicine specialist. Make an appointment so your teen can talk privately with the care provider.

Adolescence is a stage that does have risks, and some kids may be more vulnerable than others. Yet there's a lot that parents can do to keep their kids safe, make them feel loved, and help them move through the changes. Adolescence is not a disease, but a journey towards independence. It's possible for both parents and their kids to enjoy this time—and even treasure it.

Chapter 39

Child Abuse And Its Effects On Mental Health

What Is Child Abuse?[1]

Child maltreatment (or child abuse) includes all types of abuse and neglect of a child under the age of 18 by a parent, caregiver, or another person in a custodial role (e.g., clergy, coach, teacher). There are four common types of abuse.

- **Physical abuse** is the use of intentional physical force, such as hitting, kicking, shaking, burning or other show of force against a child.

- **Sexual abuse** involves engaging a child in sexual acts. It includes fondling, rape, and exposing a child to other sexual activities.

- **Emotional abuse** refers to behaviors that harm a child's self-worth or emotional well-being. Examples include name calling, shaming, rejection, withholding love, and threatening.

- **Neglect** is the failure to meet a child's basic needs. These needs include housing, food, clothing, education, and access to medical care.

Why Is Child Abuse A Public Health Problem?[2]

The few cases of abuse or neglect we see in the news are only a small part of the problem. Many cases are not reported to police or social services. What we do know is that:

- 1,640 children died in the United States in 2012 from abuse and neglect.

About This Chapter: This chapter includes text excerpted from documents published by two public domain sources. Text under the headings marked 1 are excerpted from "Understanding Child Maltreatment," Centers for Disease Control and Prevention (CDC), 2014; Text under headings marked 2 are excerpted from "Violence Prevention—Child Abuse And Neglect: Consequences," Centers for Disease Control and Prevention (CDC), March 28, 2016.

- 686,000 children were found to be victims of abuse by child protective services in 2012.

- The total lifetime economic burden resulting from new cases of fatal and nonfatal child abuse in the United States is approximately $124 billion.

How Does Child Abuse Affect Health?[1]

Child abuse has a negative effect on health. Abused children often suffer physical injuries including cuts, bruises, burns, and broken bones. In addition, abuse causes stress that can disrupt early brain development. Extreme stress can harm the development of the nervous and immune systems. As a result, children who are abused or neglected are at higher risk for health problems as adults. These problems include alcoholism, depression, drug abuse, eating disorders, obesity, high-risk sexual behaviors, smoking, suicide, and certain chronic diseases.

Child abuse and neglect may affect an individual's health and mental health in a number of direct and indirect ways. Negative effects on physical development can result from physical trauma (e.g., blows to the head or body or violent shaking) and from neglect (e.g., inadequate nutrition, lack of adequate motor stimulation, or withholding medical treatments). Abuse during infancy and early childhood has been shown to negatively affect early brain development and can have repercussions into adolescence and adulthood. The immediate emotional effects of abuse and neglect—isolation, fear, and an inability to trust—can translate into lifelong consequences including low self-esteem, depression, and relationship difficulties.

Research suggests that adults who were maltreated as children show higher rates of many health problems not typically associated with abuse and neglect, such as heart disease, cancer, chronic lung disease, and liver disease. The link between abuse and these diseases may be depression, which can influence the immune system and may lead to high-risk behaviors such as smoking, substance abuse, overeating, and sexual risk-taking.

(Source: "Health And Mental Health," Child Welfare Information Gateway, U.S. Department of Health and Human Services (HSS).)

Who Is At Risk For Child Abuse?[1]

Some factors can increase the risk for abuse or neglect. The presence of these factors does not always mean that abuse will occur. Children are never to blame for the harm others do to them.

Age. Children under 4 years of age are at greatest risk for severe injury and death from abuse.

Family environment. Abuse and neglect can occur in families where there is a great deal of stress. The stress can result from a family history of violence, drug or alcohol abuse, poverty, and chronic health problems. Families that do not have nearby friends, relatives, and other social support are also at risk.

Community. Poverty, on-going community violence, and weak connections between neighbors are related to a higher risk for child abuse and neglect.

What Are Some Of The Consequences Of Child Abuse?[2]

Child abuse and neglect affect children's health now and later, and costs to our country are significant. Neglect, physical abuse, custodial interference, and sexual abuse are types of child abuse that can lead to poor physical and mental health well into adulthood.

What Are The Effects Of Child Abuse?[2]

- Improper brain development

- Impaired cognitive (learning ability) and socio-emotional (social and emotional) skills

- Lower language development

- Blindness, cerebral palsy from head trauma

- Higher risk for heart, lung and liver diseases, obesity, cancer, high blood pressure, and high cholesterol

- Anxiety

- Smoking, alcoholism, and drug abuse

Physical

- Children may experience severe or fatal head trauma as a result of abuse. Nonfatal consequences of abusive head trauma include varying degrees of visual impairment (e.g., blindness), motor impairment (e.g., cerebral palsy) and cognitive impairments.

- Children who experience abuse and neglect are also at increased risk for adverse health effects and certain chronic diseases as adults, including heart disease, cancer, chronic lung disease, liver disease, obesity, high blood pressure, high cholesterol, and high levels of C-reactive protein.

Psychological

- In a long-term study, as many as 80 percent of young adults who had been abused met the diagnostic criteria for at least one psychiatric disorder at age 21. These young adults exhibited many problems, including depression, anxiety, eating disorders, and suicide attempts.

- The stress of chronic abuse may result in anxiety and may make victims more vulnerable to problems, such as posttraumatic stress disorder, conduct disorder, and learning, attention, and memory difficulties.

Behavioral

- Children who experience abuse and neglect are at increased risk for smoking, alcoholism, and drug abuse as adults, as well as engaging in high-risk sexual behaviors.

- Those with a history of child abuse and neglect are 1.5 times more likely to use illicit drugs, especially marijuana, in middle adulthood.

- Studies have found abused and neglected children to be at least 25 percent more likely to experience problems such as delinquency, teen pregnancy, and low academic achievement. Similarly, a longitudinal study found that physically abused children were at greater risk of being arrested as juveniles, being a teen parent, and less likely to graduate high school.

- A National Institute of Justice (NIJ) study indicated that being abused or neglected as a child increased the likelihood of arrest as a juvenile by 59 percent. Abuse and neglect also increased the likelihood of adult criminal behavior by 28 percent and violent crime by 30 percent.

- Child abuse and neglect can have a negative effect on the ability of both men and women to establish and maintain healthy intimate relationships in adulthood.

How To Prevent Child Abuse?[1]

The ultimate goal is to stop child abuse before it starts. Strategies that promote safe, stable, and nurturing relationships (SSNRs) and environments for children and families are key to protecting against abuse and other harmful childhood experiences. These prevention strategies include improving parent-child relationships by teaching positive parenting skills like good communication, appropriate discipline, and response to children's physical and emotional needs. Programs to prevent child abuse also provide parents with social support.

Chapter 40

Bullying And Youth Violence

Youth Violence

Youth violence refers to harmful behaviors that can start early and continue into young adult-hood. The young person can be a victim, an offender, or a witness to the violence.

Youth violence includes various behaviors. Some violent acts—such as bullying, slapping, or hitting—can cause more emotional harm than physical harm. Others, such as robbery and assault (with or without weapons) can lead to serious injury or even death.

(Source: "Violence Prevention—Youth Violence," Centers for Disease Control and Prevention (CDC).)

Bullying is a form of youth violence. Centers for disease control and prevention (CDC) defines bullying as any unwanted aggressive behavior(s) by another youth or group of youths who are not siblings or current dating partners that involves an observed or perceived power imbalance and is repeated multiple times or is highly likely to be repeated. Bullying may inflict harm or distress on the targeted youth including physical, psychological, social, or educational harm. Bullying can include aggression that is physical (hitting, tripping), verbal (name calling, teasing), or relational/ social (spreading rumors, leaving out of group). A young person can be a perpetrator, a victim, or both (also known as "bully/victim").

About This Chapter: Text in this chapter begins with excerpts from "Understanding Bullying," Centers for Disease Control and Prevention (CDC), 2016; Text beginning with the heading "Bullying And Children And Youth With Disabilities And Special Health Needs" is excerpted from "Bullying And Children And Youth With Disabilities And Special Health Needs," StopBullying.gov, U.S. Department of Health and Human Services (HHS), July 13, 2012. Reviewed July 2017.

Bullying can also occur through technology and is called electronic aggression or cyber-bullying. Electronic aggression is bullying that occurs through e-mail, a chat room, instant messaging, a website, text messaging, or videos or pictures posted on websites or sent through cell phones.

Why Is Bullying A Public Health Problem?

Bullying is widespread in the United States.

- In a 2015 nationwide survey, 20 percent of high school students reported being bullied on school property in the 12 months preceding the survey.

- An estimated 16 percent of high school students reported in 2015 that they were bullied electronically in the 12 months before the survey.

How Does Bullying Affect Health?

Bullying can result in social and emotional distress, physical injury, and even death. Victimized youth are at increased risk for depression, anxiety, sleep difficulties, and poor school adjustment. Youth who bully others are at increased risk for substance use, academic problems, and violence later in adolescence and adulthood. Compared to youth who only bully, or who are only victims, bully-victims suffer the most serious consequences and are at greater risk for both mental health and behavior problems.

Who Is At Risk For Bullying?

Different factors can increase a youth's risk of engaging in or experiencing bullying. However, the presence of these factors does not always mean that a young person will bully others or be bullied.

Some of the factors associated with a higher likelihood of engaging in bullying behavior include:

- Externalizing problems, such as defiant and disruptive behavior

- Harsh parenting by caregivers

- Attitudes accepting of violence

Some of the factors associated with a higher likelihood of victimization include:

- Poor peer relationships

- Low self-esteem

- Perceived by peers as different or quiet

How To Prevent Bullying

The ultimate goal is to stop bullying before it starts. Research on preventing and addressing bullying is still developing. School-based bullying prevention programs are widely implemented, but infrequently evaluated. Based on a review of the limited research on school based bullying prevention, the following program elements are promising:

- Improving supervision of students

- Using school rules and behavior management techniques in the classroom and throughout the school to detect and address bullying by providing consequences for bullying

- Having a whole school anti-bullying policy, and enforcing that policy consistently

- Promoting cooperation among different professionals and between school staff and parents

Bullying And Children And Youth With Disabilities And Special Health Needs

Children with physical, developmental, intellectual, emotional, and sensory disabilities are more likely to be bullied than their peers. Any number of factors—physical vulnerability, social skill challenges, or intolerant environments—may increase their risk. Research suggests that some children with disabilities may bully others as well.

Kids with special health needs, such as epilepsy or food allergies, may also be at higher risk of being bullied. For kids with special health needs, bullying can include making fun of kids because of their allergies or exposing them to the things they are allergic to. In these cases, bullying is not just serious; it can mean life or death.

A small but growing amount of research shows that:

- Children with attention deficit hyperactivity disorder (ADHD) are more likely than other children to be bullied. They also are somewhat more likely than others to bully their peers.

- Children with autism spectrum disorder (ASD) are at increased risk of being bullied and left out by peers. In a study of 8–17-year-olds, researchers found that children with ASD were more than three times as likely to be bullied as their peers.

- Children with epilepsy are more likely to be bullied by peers, as are children with medical conditions that affect their appearance, such as cerebral palsy, muscular dystrophy, and spina bifida. These children frequently report being called names related to their disability.

- Children with hemiplagia (paralysis of one side of their body) are more likely than other children their age to be bullied and have fewer friends.

- Children who have diabetes and are dependent on insulin may be especially vulnerable to peer bullying.

- Children who stutter may be more likely to be bullied. In one study, 83 percent of adults who stammered as children said that they were teased or bullied; 71 percent of those who had been bullied said it happened at least once a week.

Children with learning disabilities (LD) are at a greater risk of being bullied. At least one study also has found that children with LD may also be more likely than other children to bullying their peers.

Effects Of Bullying

Kids who are bullied are more likely to have:

- **Depression and anxiety**. Signs of these include increased feelings of sadness and loneliness, changes in sleep and eating patterns, and loss of interest in activities they used to enjoy. These issues may persist into adulthood.

- **Health complaints.**

- **Decreased academic achievement**—Grade point average (GPA) and standardized test scores—and school participation. They are more likely to miss, skip, or drop out of school.

Bullying, Disability Harassment, And The Law

Bullying behavior can become "disability harassment," which is prohibited under Section 504 of the *Rehabilitation Act of 1973* and Title II of the *Americans with Disabilities Act of 1990*. According to the U.S. Department of Education (ED), disability harassment is "intimidation or abusive behavior toward a student based on disability that creates a hostile environment by interfering with or denying a student's participation in or receipt of benefits, services, or opportunities in the institution's program" (U.S. Department of Education, 2000).

Disability harassment can take different forms including verbal harassment, physical threats, or threatening written statements. When a school learns that disability harassment may have occurred, the school must investigate the incident(s) promptly and respond appropriately. Disability harassment can occur in any location that is connected with school—classrooms, the cafeteria, hallways, the playground, athletic fields, or school buses. It also can occur during school-sponsored events.

Chapter 41

Teen Dating Violence

What Is Dating Violence?[1]

Dating violence is a type of intimate partner violence. It occurs between two people in a close relationship. The nature of dating violence can be physical, emotional, or sexual.

- **Physical**—This occurs when a partner is pinched, hit, shoved, slapped, punched, or kicked.

- **Psychological/Emotional**—This means threatening a partner or harming his or her sense of self-worth. Examples include name calling, shaming, bullying, embarrassing on purpose, or keeping him/her away from friends and family.

- **Sexual**—This is forcing a partner to engage in a sex act when he or she does not or cannot consent. This can be physical or nonphysical, like threatening to spread rumors if a partner refuses to have sex.

- **Stalking**—This refers to a pattern of harassing or threatening tactics that are unwanted and cause fear in the victim.

Dating violence can take place in person or electronically, such as repeated texting or posting sexual pictures of a partner online. Unhealthy relationships can start early and last a lifetime. Teens often think some behaviors, like teasing and name calling, are a "normal" part of a relationship. However, these behaviors can become abusive and develop into more serious forms of violence.

About This Chapter: This chapter includes text excerpted from documents published by two public domain sources. Text under the headings marked 1 are excerpted from "Understanding Teen Dating Violence," Centers for Disease Control and Prevention (CDC), 2016; Text under headings marked 2 are excerpted from "Teen Dating Violence," Centers for Disease Control and Prevention (CDC), July 21, 2016.

Why Is Dating Violence A Public Health Problem?[1]

Dating violence is a widespread issue that has serious long-term and short-term effects. Many teens do not report it because they are afraid to tell friends and family.

- Among high school students who dated, 21 percent of females and 10 percent of males experienced physical and/or sexual dating violence.

- Among adult victims of rape, physical violence, and/or stalking by an intimate partner, 22 percent of women and 15 percent of men first experienced some form of partner violence between 11 and 17 years of age.

Why Does Dating Violence Happen?[2]

Communicating with your partner, managing uncomfortable emotions like anger and jealousy, and treating others with respect are a few ways to keep relationships healthy and nonviolent. Teens receive messages about how to behave in relationships from peers, adults in their lives, and the media. All too often these examples suggest that violence in a relationship is normal, but violence is never acceptable. There are reasons why violence occurs.

Violence is related to certain risk factors. Risks of having unhealthy relationships increase for teens who:

- Believe that dating violence is acceptable

- Are depressed, anxious, or have other symptoms of trauma

- Display aggression towards peers or display other aggressive behaviors

- Use drugs or illegal substances

- Engage in early sexual activity and have multiple sexual partners

- Have a friend involved in dating violence

- Have conflicts with a partner

- Witness or experience violence in the home

Dating violence can be prevented when teens, families, organizations, and communities work together to implement effective prevention strategies.

How Does Dating Violence Affect Health?[1]

Dating violence can have a negative effect on health throughout life. Youth who are victims are more likely to experience symptoms of depression and anxiety, engage in unhealthy behaviors, like using tobacco, drugs, and alcohol, or exhibit antisocial behaviors, and have suicidal thoughts. Youth who are victims of dating violence in high school are at higher risk for victimization during college.

Who Is At Risk For Dating Violence?[1]

Factors that increase risk for harming a dating partner include the following:

- Belief that dating violence is acceptable

- Depression, anxiety, and other trauma symptoms

- Aggression towards peers and other aggressive behavior

- Substance use

- Early sexual activity and having multiple sexual partners

- Having a friend involved in dating violence

- Conflict with partner

- Witnessing or experiencing violence in the home

Dating violence can happen to any teen in a romantic, dating, or sexual relationship, anytime, anywhere. In a recent national survey, 1 in 10 teens reported being hit or physically hurt on purpose by a boyfriend or girlfriend at least once in the 12 months before the survey. Additionally, during the 12 months before the survey, 1 in 10 teens reported they had been kissed, touched, or physically forced to have sexual intercourse when they did not want to at least once by someone they were dating.

(Source: "Teen Dating Violence," Centers for Disease Control and Prevention (CDC).)

What Are The Consequences Of Dating Violence?[2]

As teens develop emotionally, they are heavily influenced by experiences in their relationships. Healthy relationship behaviors can have a positive effect on a teen's emotional development. Unhealthy, abusive, or violent relationships can have severe consequences and short- and long-term negative effects on a developing teen. Youth who experience dating violence are more likely to experience the following:

- Symptoms of depression and anxiety

- Engagement in unhealthy behaviors, such as tobacco and drug use, and alcohol

- Involvement in antisocial behaviors

- Thoughts about suicide

Additionally, youth who are victims of dating violence in high school are at higher risk for victimization during college.

How Can We Prevent Dating Violence?[1]

The ultimate goal is to stop dating violence before it starts. Strategies that promote healthy relationships are vital. During the preteen and teen years, young people are learning skills they need to form positive relationships with others. This is an ideal time to promote healthy relationships and prevent patterns of dating violence that can last into adulthood.

Many prevention strategies are proven to prevent or reduce dating violence. Some effective school-based programs change norms, improve problem-solving, and address dating violence in addition to other youth risk behaviors, such as substance use and sexual risk behaviors. Other programs prevent dating violence through changes to the school environment or training influential adults, like parents/caregivers and coaches, to work with youth to prevent dating violence.

Unhealthy relationships can start early and last a lifetime. Teens often think some behaviors, like teasing and name calling, are a "normal" part of a relationship. However, these behaviors can become abusive and develop into more serious forms of violence. That is why adults need to talk to teens now about the importance of developing healthy, respectful relationships.

Dating violence can have a negative effect on health throughout life. Victims of teen dating violence are more likely to experience symptoms of depression and anxiety. They might also engage in unhealthy behaviors, such as using tobacco, drugs, and alcohol. Teens who are victims in high school are at higher risk for victimization during college and in adult relationships.

(Source: "Teen Dating Violence," Centers for Disease Control and Prevention (CDC).)

Chapter 42

Cutting And Self-Harm

Self-harm, sometimes called self-injury, is when a person purposely hurts his or her own body. There are many types of self-injury, and cutting is one type that you may have heard about. If you are hurting yourself, you can learn to stop. Make sure you talk to an adult you trust.

What Are Ways People Hurt Themselves?

Some types of injury leave permanent scars or cause serious health problems, sometimes even death. These are some forms of self-injury:

- Cutting yourself (such as using a razorblade, knife, or other sharp object)

- Punching yourself or punching things (like a wall)

- Burning yourself with cigarettes, matches, or candles

- Pulling out your hair

- Poking objects into body openings

- Breaking your bones or bruising yourself

- Poisoning yourself

About This Chapter: This chapter includes text excerpted from "Cutting And Self-Harm," girlshealth.gov, Office on Women's Health (OWH), January 7, 2015.

> ## The Dangers Of Self-Injury
> Some teens think self-injury is not a big deal, but it is. Self-injury comes with many risks. For example, cutting can lead to infections, scars, and even death. Sharing tools for cutting puts a person at risk of diseases like HIV and hepatitis. Also, once you start self-injuring, it may be hard to stop. And teens who keep hurting themselves are less likely to learn how to deal with their feelings in healthy ways.

Who Hurts Themselves?

People from all different kinds of backgrounds hurt themselves. Among teens, girls may be more likely to do it than boys. People of all ages hurt themselves, too, but self-injury most often starts in the teen years. People who hurt themselves sometimes have other problems like depression, eating disorders, or drug or alcohol abuse.

Why Do Some Teens Hurt Themselves?

Some teens who hurt themselves keep their feelings bottled up inside. The physical pain then offers a sense of relief, like the feelings are getting out. Some people who hold back strong emotions begin to feel like they have no emotions, and the injury helps them at least feel something.

Some teens say that when they hurt themselves, they are trying to stop feeling painful emotions, like rage, loneliness, or hopelessness. They may injure to distract themselves from the emotional pain. Or they may be trying to feel some sense of control over what they feel.

If you are depressed, angry, or having a hard time coping, talk with an adult you trust. Remember, you have a right to be safe and happy!

If you are hurting yourself, please get help. It is possible to get past the urge to hurt yourself. There are other ways to deal with your feelings. You can talk to your parents, your doctor, or another trusted adult, like a teacher or religious leader. Therapy can help you find healthy ways to handle problems.

What Are Signs Of Self-Injury In Others?

- Having cuts, bruises, or scars
- Wearing long sleeves or pants even in hot weather

- Making excuses about injuries

- Having sharp objects around for no clear reason

How Can I Help A Friend Who Is Self-Injuring?

If you think a friend may be hurting herself, try to get your friend to talk to a trusted adult. Your friend may need professional help. A therapist can suggest ways to cope with problems without turning to self-injury. If your friend won't get help, you should talk to an adult. This is too much for you to handle alone.

What If Someone Pressures Me To Hurt Myself?

If someone pressures you to hurt yourself, think about whether you really want a friend who tries to cause you pain. Try to hang out with other people who don't treat you this way. Try to hang out with people who make you feel good about yourself.

Chapter 43

Autism Spectrum Disorder (ASD)

Autism spectrum disorder (ASD) is the name for a group of developmental disorders. ASD includes a wide range, "a spectrum," of symptoms, skills, and levels of disability.

People with ASD often have these characteristics:

- Ongoing social problems that include difficulty communicating and interacting with others

- Repetitive behaviors as well as limited interests or activities

- Symptoms that typically are recognized in the first two years of life

- Symptoms that hurt the individual's ability to function socially, at school or work, or other areas of life

Some people are mildly impaired by their symptoms, while others are severely disabled. Treatments and services can improve a person's symptoms and ability to function. Families with concerns should talk to their pediatrician about what they've observed and the possibility of ASD screening. According to the Centers for Disease Control and Prevention (CDC) around 1 in 68 children has been identified with some form of ASD.

Signs And Symptoms Of Autism Spectrum Disorder (ASD)

Parents or doctors may first identify ASD behaviors in infants and toddlers. School staff may recognize these behaviors in older children. Not all people with ASD will show all of these behaviors, but most will show several.

About This Chapter: This chapter includes text excerpted from "Autism Spectrum Disorder," National Institute of Mental Health (NIMH), October 2016.

There are two main types of behaviors: "restricted/repetitive behaviors" and "social communication/interaction behaviors."

1. Restrictive/repetitive behaviors may include:

- Repeating certain behaviors or having unusual behaviors

- Having overly focused interests, such as with moving objects or parts of objects

- Having a lasting, intense interest in certain topics, such as numbers, details, or facts.

2. Social communication/interaction behaviors may include:

- Getting upset by a slight change in a routine or being placed in a new or overly stimulating setting

- Making little or inconsistent eye contact

- Having a tendency to look at and listen to other people less often

- Rarely sharing enjoyment of objects or activities by pointing or showing things to others

- Responding in an unusual way when others show anger, distress, or affection

- Failing to, or being slow to, respond to someone calling their name or other verbal attempts to gain attention

- Having difficulties with the back and forth of conversations

- Often talking at length about a favorite subject without noticing that others are not interested or without giving others a chance to respond

- Repeating words or phrases that they hear, a behavior called echolalia

- Using words that seem odd, out of place, or have a special meaning known only to those familiar with that person's way of communicating

- Having facial expressions, movements, and gestures that do not match what is being said

- Having an unusual tone of voice that may sound sing-song or flat and robot-like

- Having trouble understanding another person's point of view or being unable to predict or understand other people's actions.

People with ASD may have other difficulties, such as being very sensitive to light, noise, clothing, or temperature. They may also experience sleep problems, digestion problems, and irritability. ASD is unique in that it is common for people with ASD to have many strengths and abilities in addition to challenges.

Strengths and abilities may include:

- Having above-average intelligence—the CDC reports 46 percent of ASD children have above average intelligence

- Being able to learn things in detail and remember information for long periods of time

- Being strong visual and auditory learners

- Excelling in math, science, music, or art.

Risk Factors Of ASD

Scientists don't know the exact causes of ASD, but research suggests that genes and environment play important roles.

Risk factors include:

- Gender—boys are more likely to be diagnosed with ASD than girls

- Having a sibling with ASD

- Having older parents (a mother who was 35 or older, and/or a father who was 40 or older when the baby was born)

- Genetics—about 20 percent of children with ASD also have certain genetic conditions. Those conditions include Down syndrome, fragile X syndrome, and tuberous sclerosis among others.

In recent years, the number of children identified with ASD has increased. Experts disagree about whether this shows a true increase in ASD since the guidelines for diagnosis have changed in recent years as well. Also, many more parents and doctors now know about the disorder, so parents are more likely to have their children screened, and more doctors are able to properly diagnose ASD, even in adulthood.

Diagnosing ASD

Doctors diagnose ASD by looking at a child's behavior and development. Young children with ASD can usually be reliably diagnosed by age two. Older children and adolescents should be evaluated for ASD when a parent or teacher raises concerns based on watching the child socialize, communicate, and play.

Diagnosis In Young Children

Diagnosis in young children is often a two-stage process:

Stage 1: General Developmental Screening During Well-Child Checkups

Every child should receive well-child check-ups with a pediatrician or an early childhood healthcare provider. The Centers for Disease Control and Prevention (CDC) recommends specific ASD screening be done at the 18- and 24-month visits.

Earlier screening might be needed if a child is at high risk for ASD or developmental problems. Those at high risk include children who:

- Have a sister, brother, or other family member with ASD

- Have some ASD behaviors

- Were born premature, or early, and at a low birth weight.

Parents' experiences and concerns are very important in the screening process for young children. Sometimes the doctor will ask parents questions about the child's behaviors and combine this information with his or her observations of the child. Children who show some developmental problems during this screening process will be referred for another stage of evaluation.

Stage 2: Additional Evaluation

This evaluation is with a team of doctors and other health professionals with a wide range of specialties who are experienced in diagnosing ASD. This team may include:

- A developmental pediatrician—a doctor who has special training in child development

- A child psychologist and/or child psychiatrist—a doctor who knows about brain development and behavior

- A speech-language pathologist—a health professional who has special training in communication difficulties.

The evaluation may assess:

- Cognitive level or thinking skills

- Language abilities

- Age-appropriate skills needed to complete daily activities independently, such as eating, dressing, and toileting.

Because ASD is a complex disorder that sometimes occurs along with other illnesses or learning disorders, the comprehensive evaluation may include:

- Blood tests

- Hearing test

The outcome of the evaluation will result in recommendations to help plan for treatment.

Diagnosis In Older Children And Adolescents

Older children whose ASD symptoms are noticed after starting school are often first recognized and evaluated by the school's special education team. The school's team may refer these children to a healthcare professional.

Parents may talk with a pediatrician about their child's social difficulties including problems with subtle communication. These subtle communication issues may include understanding tone of voice, facial expressions, or body language. Older children may have trouble understanding figures of speech, humor, or sarcasm. Parents may also find that their child has trouble forming friendships with peers. The pediatrician can refer the child for further evaluation and treatment.

Treatments And Therapies For ASD

Early treatment for ASD and proper care can reduce individuals' difficulties while helping them learn new skills and make the most of their strengths. The very wide range of issues facing those "on the spectrum" means that there is no single best treatment for ASD. Working closely with a doctor or healthcare professional is an important part of finding the right treatment program. There are many treatment options, social services, programs, and other resources that can help.

Here are some tips.

- Keep a detailed notebook. Record conversations and meetings with healthcare providers and teachers. This information helps when it's time to make decisions.

- Record doctors' reports and evaluations in the notebook. This information may help an individual qualify for special programs.

- Contact the local health department, school, or autism advocacy groups to learn about their special programs.

- Talk with a pediatrician, school official, or physician to find a local autism expert who can help develop an intervention plan and find other local resources.

- Find an autism support group. Sharing information and experiences can help individuals with ASD and/or their caregivers learn about options, make decisions, and reduce stress.

Medication

A doctor may use medication to treat some difficulties that are common with ASD. With medication, a person with ASD may have fewer problems with:

- Irritability

- Aggression

- Repetitive behavior

- Hyperactivity

- Attention problems

- Anxiety and depression

Medications might not affect all children in the same way. It is important to work with a healthcare professional who has experience in treating children with ASD. Parents and healthcare professionals must closely monitor a child's progress and reactions while he or she is taking a medication to be sure that any negative side effects of the treatment do not outweigh the benefits.

It is also important to remember that children with ASD can get sick or injured just like children without ASD. Regular medical and dental exams should be part of a child's treatment plan. Often it is hard to tell if a child's behavior is related to the ASD or is caused by a separate health condition. For instance, head banging could be a symptom of the ASD, or it could be a sign that the child is having headaches. In those cases, a thorough physical exam is needed. Monitoring healthy development means not only paying attention to symptoms related to ASD, but also to the child's physical and mental health, as well.

(Source: "Autism Spectrum Disorder—Treatment," Centers for Disease Control and Prevention (CDC).)

Chapter 44

Attention Deficit Hyperactivity Disorder

Do you find it hard to pay attention? Do you feel the need to move constantly during times when you shouldn't? Do you find yourself constantly interrupting others? If these issues are ongoing and you feel that they are negatively impacting your daily life, it could be a sign of attention deficit hyperactivity disorder (ADHD).

ADHD is a disorder that makes it difficult for a person to pay attention and control impulsive behaviors. He or she may also be restless and almost constantly active.

ADHD is not just a childhood disorder. Although the symptoms of ADHD begin in childhood, ADHD can continue through adolescence and adulthood. Even though hyperactivity tends to improve as a child becomes a teen, problems with inattention, disorganization, and poor impulse control often continue through the teen years and into adulthood.

(Source: "Attention Deficit Hyperactivity Disorder: The Basics," National Institute of Mental Health (NIMH).)

ADHD is a brain disorder marked by an ongoing pattern of inattention and/or hyperactivity-impulsivity that interferes with functioning or development.

- **Inattention** means a person wanders off task, lacks persistence, has difficulty sustaining focus, and is disorganized; and these problems are not due to defiance or lack of comprehension.

- **Hyperactivity** means a person seems to move about constantly, including in situations in which it is not appropriate; or excessively fidgets, taps, or talks. In adults, it may be extreme restlessness or wearing others out with constant activity.

About This Chapter: This chapter includes text excerpted from "Attention Deficit Hyperactivity Disorder," National Institute of Mental Health (NIMH), March 2016.

- **Impulsivity** means a person makes hasty actions that occur in the moment without first thinking about them and that may have high potential for harm; or a desire for immediate rewards or inability to delay gratification. An impulsive person may be socially intrusive and excessively interrupt others or make important decisions without considering the long-term consequences.

Signs And Symptoms Of Attention Deficit Hyperactivity Disorder (ADHD)

Inattention and hyperactivity/impulsivity are the key behaviors of ADHD. Some people with ADHD only have problems with one of the behaviors, while others have both inattention and hyperactivity-impulsivity. Most children have the combined type of ADHD. In preschool, the most common ADHD symptom is hyperactivity. It is normal to have some inattention, unfocused motor activity and impulsivity, but for people with ADHD, these behaviors:

- are more severe

- occur more often

- interfere with or reduce the quality of how they functions socially, at school, or in a job

Inattention

People with symptoms of inattention may often:

- Overlook or miss details, make careless mistakes in schoolwork, at work, or during other activities

- Have problems sustaining attention in tasks or play, including conversations, lectures, or lengthy reading

- Not seem to listen when spoken to directly

- Not follow through on instructions and fail to finish schoolwork, chores, or duties in the workplace or start tasks but quickly lose focus and get easily sidetracked

- Have problems organizing tasks and activities, such as what to do in sequence, keeping materials and belongings in order, having messy work and poor time management, and failing to meet deadlines

- Avoid or dislike tasks that require sustained mental effort, such as schoolwork or homework, or for teens and older adults, preparing reports, completing forms or reviewing lengthy papers

- Lose things necessary for tasks or activities, such as school supplies, pencils, books, tools, wallets, keys, paperwork, eyeglasses, and cell phones

- Be easily distracted by unrelated thoughts or stimuli

- Be forgetful in daily activities, such as chores, errands, returning calls, and keeping appointments

Hyperactivity-Impulsivity

People with symptoms of hyperactivity-impulsivity may often:

- Fidget and squirm in their seats

- Leave their seats in situations when staying seated is expected, such as in the classroom or in the office

- Run or dash around or climb in situations where it is inappropriate or, in teens and adults, often feel restless

- Be unable to play or engage in hobbies quietly

- Be constantly in motion or "on the go," or act as if "driven by a motor"

- Talk nonstop

- Blurt out an answer before a question has been completed, finish other people's sentences, or speak without waiting for a turn in conversation

- Have trouble waiting his or her turn

- Interrupt or intrude on others, for example in conversations, games, or activities

Diagnosis Of ADHD

Diagnosis of ADHD requires a comprehensive evaluation by a licensed clinician, such as a pediatrician, psychologist, or psychiatrist with expertise in ADHD. For a person to receive a diagnosis of ADHD, the symptoms of inattention and/or hyperactivity-impulsivity must be chronic or long-lasting, impair the person's functioning, and cause the person to fall behind normal development for his or her age. The doctor will also ensure that any ADHD symptoms are not due to another medical or psychiatric condition. Most children with ADHD receive a diagnosis during the elementary school years. For an adolescent or adult to receive a diagnosis of ADHD, the symptoms need to have been present prior to age 12.

ADHD symptoms can appear as early as between the ages of 3 and 6 and can continue through adolescence and adulthood. Symptoms of ADHD can be mistaken for emotional or disciplinary problems or missed entirely in quiet, well-behaved children, leading to a delay in diagnosis. Adults with undiagnosed ADHD may have a history of poor academic performance, problems at work, or difficult or failed relationships.

ADHD symptoms can change over time as a person ages.

In young children with ADHD, hyperactivity-impulsivity is the most predominant symptom. As a child reaches elementary school, the symptom of inattention may become more prominent and cause the child to struggle academically. In adolescence, hyperactivity seems to lessen and may show more often as feelings of restlessness or fidgeting, but inattention and impulsivity may remain. Many adolescents with ADHD also struggle with relationships and antisocial behaviors. Inattention, restlessness, and impulsivity tend to persist into adulthood.

Risk Factors Of ADHD

Scientists are not sure what causes ADHD. Like many other illnesses, a number of factors can contribute to ADHD, such as:

- Genes

- Cigarette smoking, alcohol use, or drug use during pregnancy

- Exposure to environmental toxins during pregnancy

- Exposure to environmental toxins, such as high levels of lead, at a young age

- Low birth weight

- Brain injuries

ADHD is more common in males than females, and females with ADHD are more likely to have problems primarily with inattention. Other conditions, such as learning disabilities, anxiety disorder, conduct disorder, depression, and substance abuse, are common in people with ADHD.

Treatment And Therapies Of ADHD

While there is no cure for ADHD, currently available treatments can help reduce symptoms and improve functioning. Treatments include medication, psychotherapy, education or training, or a combination of treatments.

Medication

For many people, ADHD medications reduce hyperactivity and impulsivity and improve their ability to focus, work, and learn. Medication also may improve physical coordination. Sometimes several different medications or dosages must be tried before finding the right one that works for a particular person. Anyone taking medications must be monitored closely and carefully by their prescribing doctor.

Stimulants. The most common type of medication used for treating ADHD is called a "stimulant." Although it may seem unusual to treat ADHD with a medication that is considered a stimulant, it works because it increases the brain chemicals dopamine and norepinephrine, which play essential roles in thinking and attention.

Under medical supervision, stimulant medications are considered safe. However, there are risks and side effects, especially when misused or taken in excess of the prescribed dose. For example, stimulants can raise blood pressure and heart rate and increase anxiety. Therefore, a person with other health problems, including high blood pressure, seizures, heart disease, glaucoma, liver or kidney disease, or an anxiety disorder should tell their doctor before taking a stimulant.

Talk with a doctor if you see any of these side effects while taking stimulants:

- decreased appetite

- sleep problems

- tics (sudden, repetitive movements or sounds)

- personality changes

- increased anxiety and irritability

- stomachaches

- headaches

Nonstimulants. A few other ADHD medications are nonstimulants. These medications take longer to start working than stimulants, but can also improve focus, attention, and impulsivity in a person with ADHD. Doctors may prescribe a nonstimulant: when a person has bothersome side effects from stimulants; when a stimulant was not effective; or in combination with a stimulant to increase effectiveness.

Although not approved by the U.S. Food and Drug Administration (FDA) specifically for the treatment of ADHD, some antidepressants are sometimes used alone or in combination with a stimulant to treat ADHD. Antidepressants may help all of the symptoms of ADHD and can be prescribed if a patient has bothersome side effects from stimulants. Antidepressants can be helpful in combination with stimulants if a patient also has another condition, such as an anxiety disorder, depression, or another mood disorder.

Doctors and patients can work together to find the best medication, dose, or medication combination.

Psychotherapy

Adding psychotherapy to treat ADHD can help patients and their families to better cope with everyday problems.

Behavioral therapy is a type of psychotherapy that aims to help a person change his or her behavior. It might involve practical assistance, such as help organizing tasks or completing schoolwork, or working through emotionally difficult events. Behavioral therapy also teaches a person how to:

- monitor his or her own behavior

- give oneself praise or rewards for acting in a desired way, such as controlling anger or thinking before acting

Parents, teachers, and family members also can give positive or negative feedback for certain behaviors and help establish clear rules, chore lists, and other structured routines to help a person control his or her behavior. Therapists may also teach children social skills, such as how to wait their turn, share toys, ask for help, or respond to teasing. Learning to read facial expressions and the tone of voice in others, and how to respond appropriately can also be part of social skills training.

Cognitive behavioral therapy can also teach a person mindfulness techniques, or meditation. A person learns how to be aware and accepting of one's own thoughts and feelings to improve focus and concentration. The therapist also encourages the person with ADHD to adjust to the life changes that come with treatment, such as thinking before acting, or resisting the urge to take unnecessary risks.

Family and marital therapy can help family members and spouses find better ways to handle disruptive behaviors, to encourage behavior changes, and improve interactions with the patient.

Education And Training For ADHD Patients

Children with ADHD need guidance and understanding from their parents, families, and teachers to reach their full potential and to succeed. For school-age children, frustration, blame, and anger may have built up within a family before a child is diagnosed. Parents and children may need special help to overcome negative feelings. Mental health professionals can educate parents about ADHD and how it affects a family. They also will help the child and his or her parents develop new skills, attitudes, and ways of relating to each other.

Parenting skills training (behavioral parent management training) teaches parents the skills they need to encourage and reward positive behaviors in their children. It helps parents learn how to use a system of rewards and consequences to change a child's behavior. Parents are taught to give immediate and positive feedback for behaviors they want to encourage, and ignore or redirect behaviors that they want to discourage. They may also learn to structure situations in ways that support desired behavior.

Stress management techniques can benefit parents of children with ADHD by increasing their ability to deal with frustration so that they can respond calmly to their child's behavior.

Support groups can help parents and families connect with others who have similar problems and concerns. Groups often meet regularly to share frustrations and successes, to exchange information about recommended specialists and strategies, and to talk with experts.

Tips To Help Kids With ADHD Stay Organized

Parents and teachers can help kids with ADHD stay organized and follow directions with tools such as:

- Keeping a routine and a schedule. Keep the same routine every day, from wake-up time to bedtime. Include times for homework, outdoor play, and indoor activities. Keep the schedule on the refrigerator or on a bulletin board in the kitchen. Write changes on the schedule as far in advance as possible.

- Organizing everyday items. Have a place for everything, and keep everything in its place. This includes clothing, backpacks, and toys.

- Using homework and notebook organizers. Use organizers for school material and supplies. Stress to your child the importance of writing down assignments and bringing home the necessary books.

- Being clear and consistent. Children with ADHD need consistent rules they can understand and follow.

- Giving praise or rewards when rules are followed. Children with ADHD often receive and expect criticism. Look for good behavior, and praise it.

Chapter 45

Tourette Syndrome And Tics

Tourette syndrome (TS) is a condition of the nervous system. TS causes people to have "tics." Tics are sudden twitches, movements, or sounds that people do repeatedly. People who have tics cannot stop their body from doing these things.

For example, a person might keep blinking over and over again. Or, a person might make a grunting sound unwillingly. Having tics is a little bit like having hiccups. Even though you might not want to hiccup, your body does it anyway. Sometimes people can stop themselves from doing a certain tic for awhile, but it's hard. Eventually the person has to do the tic.

Types Of Tics

There are two types of tics—motor and vocal:

1. Motor Tics

Motor tics are movements of the body. Examples of motor tics include blinking, shrugging the shoulders, or jerking an arm.

2. Vocal Tics

Vocal tics are sounds that a person makes with his or her voice. Examples of vocal tics include humming, clearing the throat, or yelling out a word or phrase.

About This Chapter: This chapter includes text excerpted from "Facts About Tourette Syndrome," Centers for Disease Control and Prevention (CDC), May 11, 2017.

Tics can be either simple or complex:

Simple Tics

Simple tics involve just a few parts of the body. Examples of simple tics include squinting the eyes or sniffing.

Complex Tics

Complex tics usually involve several different parts of the body and can have a pattern. An example of a complex tic is bobbing the head while jerking an arm, and then jumping up.

Symptoms Of Tourette Syndrome (TS)

The main symptoms of TS are tics. Symptoms usually begin when a child is 5 to 10 years of age. The first symptoms often are motor tics that occur in the head and neck area. Tics usually are worse during times that are stressful or exciting. They tend to improve when a person is calm or focused on an activity. The types of tics and how often a person has tics changes a lot over time. Even though the symptoms might appear, disappear, and reappear, these conditions are considered chronic.

In most cases, tics decrease during adolescence and early adulthood, and sometimes disappear entirely. However, many people with TS experience tics into adulthood and, in some cases, tics can become worse during adulthood. Although the media often portray people with TS as involuntarily shouting out swear words (called coprolalia) or constantly repeating the words of other people (called echolalia), these symptoms are rare, and are not required for a diagnosis of TS.

Risk Factors And Causes Of TS

Doctors and scientists do not know the exact cause of TS. Research suggests that it is an inherited genetic condition. That means it is passed on from parent to child through *genes*. Scientists are studying the causes of and risk factors for TS in an effort to understand it better, and to find better ways to manage TS and to reduce the chances of a person having TS. The causes of TS and other tic disorders are not well understood.

Although the risk factors for and causes of TS are unknown, current research shows that genes play an important role:

- Genetic studies have indicated that TS is inherited as a dominant gene, with about a 50 percent chance of parents passing the gene on to their children.

- Boys with the gene(s) are three to four times more likely than girls to display symptoms of TS.

- TS can be triggered by abnormal metabolism (breakdown) of a chemical in the brain called dopamine.

Some research has shown that TS is a genetically complex disorder that likely occurs as a result of the effects of multiple genes interacting with other factors in the environment. Scientists are studying other possible causes and environmental risk factors that might contribute to TS. Some studies have shown that the following factors might be associated with TS, but additional research is needed to better understand these associations:

- Mother drinking alcohol or smoking during pregnancy.

- Complications during birth.

- Low birthweight.

- **Infection.** Researchers are investigating whether certain children are more likely to develop tics following a group A ß-hemolytic streptococcal ("strep") infection. This is referred to as Pediatric Autoimmune Neuropsychiatric Disorders Associated with Streptococcal (PANDAS) infections.

Diagnosis Of TS

There is no single test, like a blood test, to diagnose TS. Health professionals look at the person's symptoms to diagnose TS and other tic disorders. The tic disorders differ from each other in terms of the type of tic present (motor or vocal, or combination of the both), and how long the symptoms have lasted. TS can be diagnosed if a person has both motor and vocal tics, and has had tic symptoms for at least a year.

The American Psychiatric Association's (APA) *Diagnostic and Statistical Manual of Mental Disorders, Fifth Edition* (DSM-5) is used by health professionals to help diagnose tic disorders.

Tics are sudden twitches, movements, or sounds that people do repeatedly. People who have tics cannot stop their body from doing these things. For example, a person with a motor tic might keep blinking over and over again. Or, a person with a vocal tic might make a grunting sound unwillingly.

Three tic disorders are included in the DSM-5:

- Tourette's disorder (also called Tourette syndrome [TS])

- Persistent (also called chronic) motor or vocal tic disorder

- Provisional tic disorder

The tic disorders differ from each other in terms of the type of tic present (motor or vocal, or a combination of both), and how long the symptoms have lasted. People with TS have both motor and vocal tics, and have had tic symptoms for at least 1 year. People with persistent motor or vocal tic disorders have either motor or vocal tics, and have had tic symptoms for at least 1 year. People with provisional tic disorders can have motor or vocal tics, or both, but have had their symptoms less than 1 year.

Treatments Of TS

Although there is no cure for TS, there are treatments available to help manage the tics. Many people with TS have tics that do not get in the way of their daily life and, therefore, do not need any treatment. However, medication and behavioral treatments are available if tics cause pain or injury; interfere with school, work, or social life; or cause stress.

Although there is no cure for Tourette Syndrome (TS), there are treatments to help manage the tics caused by TS. Many people with TS have tics that do not get in the way of their living their daily life and, therefore, do not need any treatment. However, medication and behavioral treatments are available if tics cause pain or injury; interfere with school, work, or social life; or cause stress. A promising new behavioral treatment is the Comprehensive Behavioral Intervention for Tics (CBIT)

Educating the community (for example, peers, educators, and coworkers) about TS can increase understanding of the symptoms, reduce teasing, and decrease stress for people living with TS. People with TS cannot help having tics, and are not being disruptive on purpose. When others understand these facts, people with TS might receive more support, which might, in turn, help lessen some tic symptoms.

It is common for people with TS to have cooccurring conditions, particularly attention deficit hyperactivity disorder (ADHD) and obsessive-compulsive disorder (OCD). People with additional conditions will require different treatments based on the symptoms. Sometimes treating these other conditions can help reduce tics. To develop the best treatment plan, people with tics, parents, and healthcare providers should work closely with one another, and with everyone involved in treatment and support—which may include teachers, child care providers, coaches, therapists, and other family members. Taking advantage of all the resources available will help guide success.

Medications

Medications can be used to reduce severe or disruptive tics that might have led to problems in the past with family and friends, other students, or coworkers. Medications also can be used to reduce symptoms of related conditions, such as ADHD or OCD.

Medications do not eliminate tics completely. However, they can help some people with TS in their everyday life. There is no one medication that is best for all people. Most medications prescribed for TS have not been approved by the U.S. Food and Drug Administration (FDA) for treating tics.

Medications affect each person differently. One person might do well with one medication, but not another. When deciding the best treatment, a doctor might try different medications and doses, and it may take time to find the treatment plan that works best. The doctor will want to find the medication and dose that have the best results and the fewest side effects. Doctors often start with small doses and slowly increase as needed.

As with all medications, those used to treat tics can have side effects. Side effects can include weight gain, stiff muscles, tiredness, restlessness, and social withdrawal. The side effects need to be considered carefully when deciding whether or not to use any medication to treat tics. In some cases, the side effects can be worse than the tics.

Even though medications often are used to treat the symptoms of TS, they might not be helpful for everyone. Two common reasons for not using medications to treat TS are unpleasant side effects and failure of the medications to work as well as expected.

Behavioral Therapy

Behavioral therapy is a treatment that teaches people with TS ways to manage their tics. Behavioral therapy is not a cure for tics. However, it can help reduce the number of tics, the severity of tics, the impact of tics, or a combination of all of these. It is important to understand that even though behavioral therapies might help reduce the severity of tics, this does not mean that tics are just psychological or that anyone with tics should be able to control them.

Habit Reversal

Habit reversal is one of the most studied behavioral interventions for people with tics. It has two main parts: awareness training and competing response training. In the awareness training part, people identify each tic out loud. In the competing response part, people learn to do a new behavior that cannot happen at the same time as the tic. For example, if the person

247

with TS has a tic that involves head rubbing, a new behavior might be for that person to place his or her hands on his or her knees, or to cross his or her arms so that the head rubbing cannot take place.

Comprehensive Behavioral Intervention For Tics (CBIT)

CBIT is a new, evidence-based type of behavioral therapy for TS and chronic tic disorders. CBIT includes habit reversal in addition to other strategies, including education about tics and relaxation techniques. CBIT has been shown to be effective at reducing tic symptoms and tic-related impairment among children and adults.

In CBIT, a therapist will work with a child (and his or her parents) or an adult with TS to better understand the types of tics the person is having and to understand the situations in which the tics are at their worst. Changes to the surroundings may be made, if possible, and the person with TS will also learn to do a new behavior instead of the tic (habit reversal). For example, if a child with TS often has a certain tic during math class, the math teacher can be educated about TS, and perhaps the child's seat can be changed so that the tics are not as visible. In addition, the child also can work with a psychologist to learn habit reversal techniques. This helps to decrease how often the tic occurs by doing a new behavior (like putting his or her hands on his or her knees when an urge to perform the tic happens). CBIT skills can be learned with practice, with the help of an experienced therapist, and with the support and encouragement of those close to the person with TS.

In recent years, more health professionals have recognized that behavioral therapy can be very effective in managing the symptoms of TS. Unfortunately, very few clinicians have been trained in these types of treatments specifically for TS and tic disorders. The Centers for Disease Control and Prevention (CDC) and The Tourette Association of America have been working to educate more health professionals in this approach to managing TS symptoms.

Chapter 46

Depression During And After Pregnancy

What Is Depression?

Depression is more than just feeling "blue" or "down in the dumps" for a few days. It's a serious illness that involves the brain. With depression, sad, anxious, or "empty" feelings don't go away and interfere with day-to-day life and routines. These feelings can be mild to severe. The good news is that most people with depression get better with treatment.

How Common Is Depression During And After Pregnancy

Depression is a common problem during and after pregnancy. About 13 percent of pregnant women and new mothers have depression.

As many as 1 in 9 women experience depression before, during, or after pregnancy.

(Source: "Maternal Depression," Centers for Disease Control and Prevention (CDC).)

Approximately 4 percent of fathers experience depression in the first year after their child's birth. By a child's 12th birthday, about 1 out of 5 fathers will have experienced one or more episodes of depression. Younger fathers, those with a history of depression, and those experiencing difficulties affording items such as a home or car were most likely to experience depression.

(Source: "Depression Among Women," Centers for Disease Control and Prevention (CDC).)

About This Chapter: This chapter includes text excerpted from "Depression During And After Pregnancy Fact Sheet," Office on Women's Health (OWH), U.S. Department of Health and Human Services (HHS), February 12, 2016.

How Do I Know If I Have Depression?

When you are pregnant or after you have a baby, you may be depressed and not know it. Some normal changes during and after pregnancy can cause symptoms similar to those of depression. But if you have any of the following symptoms of depression for more than 2 weeks, call your doctor:

- Feeling restless or moody

- Feeling sad, hopeless, and overwhelmed

- Crying a lot

- Having no energy or motivation

- Eating too little or too much

- Sleeping too little or too much

- Having trouble focusing or making decisions

- Having memory problems

- Feeling worthless and guilty

- Losing interest or pleasure in activities you used to enjoy

- Withdrawing from friends and family

- Having headaches, aches and pains, or stomach problems that don't go away

Your doctor can figure out if your symptoms are caused by depression or something else.

What Causes Depression? What About Postpartum Depression?

There is no single cause. Rather, depression likely results from a combination of factors:

- Depression is a mental illness that tends to run in families. Women with a family history of depression are more likely to have depression.

- Changes in brain chemistry or structure are believed to play a big role in depression.

- Stressful life events, such as death of a loved one, caring for an aging family member, abuse, and poverty, can trigger depression.

- Hormonal factors unique to women may contribute to depression in some women. We know that hormones directly affect the brain chemistry that controls emotions and mood. We also know that women are at greater risk of depression at certain times in their lives, such as puberty, during and after pregnancy, and during perimenopause. Some women also have depressive symptoms right before their period.

Depression after childbirth is called postpartum depression. Hormonal changes may trigger symptoms of postpartum depression. When you are pregnant, levels of the female hormones estrogen and progesterone increase greatly. In the first 24 hours after childbirth, hormone levels quickly return to normal. Researchers think the big change in hormone levels may lead to depression. This is much like the way smaller hormone changes can affect a woman's moods before she gets her period.

Levels of thyroid hormones may also drop after giving birth. The thyroid is a small gland in the neck that helps regulate how your body uses and stores energy from food. Low levels of thyroid hormones can cause symptoms of depression. A simple blood test can tell if this condition is causing your symptoms. If so, your doctor can prescribe thyroid medicine.

Other factors may play a role in postpartum depression. You may feel:

*   Tired after delivery
*   Tired from a lack of sleep or broken sleep
*   Overwhelmed with a new baby
*   Doubts about your ability to be a good mother
*   Stress from changes in work and home routines
*   An unrealistic need to be a perfect mom
*   Loss of who you were before having the baby
*   Less attractive
*   A lack of free time

Are Some Women More At Risk For Depression During And After Pregnancy?

Certain factors may increase your risk of depression during and after pregnancy:

*   A personal history of depression or another mental illness
*   A family history of depression or another mental illness
*   A lack of support from family and friends

- Anxiety or negative feelings about the pregnancy

- Problems with a previous pregnancy or birth

- Marriage or money problems

- Stressful life events

- Young age

- Substance abuse

Women who are depressed during pregnancy have a greater risk of depression after giving birth. The U.S. Preventive Services Task Force (USPSTF) recommends screening for depression during and after pregnancy, regardless of a woman's risk factors for depression.

What Is The Difference Between "Baby Blues," Postpartum Depression, And Postpartum Psychosis?

Many women have the baby blues in the days after childbirth. If you have the baby blues, you may:

- Have mood swings

- Feel sad, anxious, or overwhelmed

- Have crying spells

- Lose your appetite

- Have trouble sleeping

The baby blues most often go away within a few days or a week. The symptoms are not severe and do not need treatment.

The symptoms of postpartum depression last longer and are more severe. Postpartum depression can begin anytime within the first year after childbirth. If you have postpartum depression, you may have any of the symptoms of depression listed above. Symptoms may also include:

- Thoughts of hurting the baby

- Thoughts of hurting yourself

- Not having any interest in the baby

Postpartum depression needs to be treated by a doctor.

Postpartum psychosis is rare. It occurs in about 1 to 4 out of every 1,000 births. It usually begins in the first 2 weeks after childbirth. Women who have bipolar disorder or another mental health problem called schizoaffective disorder have a higher risk for postpartum psychosis. Symptoms may include:

- Seeing things that aren't there

- Feeling confused

- Having rapid mood swings

- Trying to hurt yourself or your baby

What Should I Do If I Have Symptoms Of Depression During Or After Pregnancy?

Call your doctor if:

- Your baby blues don't go away after 2 weeks

- Symptoms of depression get more and more intense

- Symptoms of depression begin any time after delivery, even many months later

- It is hard for you to perform tasks at work or at home

- You cannot care for yourself or your baby

- You have thoughts of harming yourself or your baby

Your doctor can ask you questions to test for depression. Your doctor can also refer you to a mental health professional who specializes in treating depression.

Some women don't tell anyone about their symptoms. They feel embarrassed, ashamed, or guilty about feeling depressed when they are supposed to be happy. They worry they will be viewed as unfit parents.

Any woman may become depressed during pregnancy or after having a baby. It doesn't mean you are a bad or "not together" mom. You and your baby don't have to suffer. There is help.

Here are some other helpful tips:

- Rest as much as you can. Sleep when the baby is sleeping.

- Don't try to do too much or try to be perfect.

- Ask your partner, family, and friends for help.

- Make time to go out, visit friends, or spend time alone with your partner.

- Discuss your feelings with your partner, family, and friends.

- Talk with other mothers so you can learn from their experiences.

- Join a support group. Ask your doctor about groups in your area.

- Don't make any major life changes during pregnancy or right after giving birth. Major changes can cause unneeded stress. Sometimes big changes can't be avoided. When that happens, try to arrange support and help in your new situation ahead of time.

How Is Depression Treated?

The two common types of treatment for depression are:

1. **Talk therapy.** This involves talking to a therapist, psychologist, or social worker to learn to change how depression makes you think, feel, and act.

2. **Medicine.** Your doctor can prescribe an antidepressant medicine. These medicines can help relieve symptoms of depression.

These treatment methods can be used alone or together. If you are depressed, your depression can affect your baby. Getting treatment is important for you and your baby. Talk with your doctor about the benefits and risks of taking medicine to treat depression when you are pregnant or breastfeeding.

Did You Know?
If you take medicine for depression, stopping your medicine when you become pregnant can cause your depression to come back. Do not stop any prescribed medicines without first talking to your doctor. Not using medicine that you need may be harmful to you or your baby.

What Can Happen If Depression Is Not Treated?

Untreated depression can hurt you and your baby. Some women with depression have a hard time caring for themselves during pregnancy. They may:

- Eat poorly

- Not gain enough weight

- Have trouble sleeping

- Miss prenatal visits

- Not follow medical instructions

- Use harmful substances, like tobacco, alcohol, or illegal drugs

Depression during pregnancy can raise the risk of:

- Problems during pregnancy or delivery

- Having a low-birth-weight baby

- Premature birth

Untreated postpartum depression can affect your ability to parent. You may:

- Lack energy

- Have trouble focusing

- Feel moody

- Not be able to meet your child's needs

As a result, you may feel guilty and lose confidence in yourself as a mother. These feelings can make your depression worse.

Researchers believe postpartum depression in a mother can affect her baby. It can cause the baby to have:

- Delays in language development

- Problems with mother-child bonding

- Behavior problems

- Increased crying

It helps if your partner or another caregiver can help meet the baby's needs while you are depressed.

All children deserve the chance to have a healthy mom. And all moms deserve the chance to enjoy their life and their children. If you are feeling depressed during pregnancy or after having a baby, don't suffer alone. Please tell a loved one and call your doctor right away.

Part Six
Mental Health Treatments

Chapter 47

Diagnosing Mental Illness

Research shows that half of all lifetime cases of mental illness begin by age 14. Scientists are discovering that changes in the body leading to mental illness may start much earlier, before any symptoms appear. Through greater understanding of when and how fast specific areas of children's brains develop, we are learning more about the early stages of a wide range of mental illnesses that appear later in life. Helping young children and their parents manage difficulties early in life may prevent the development of disorders. Once mental illness develops, it becomes a regular part of the child's behavior and more difficult to treat.

Even though we know how to treat (though not yet cure) many disorders, many children with mental illnesses are not getting treatment. This chapter addresses common questions about diagnosis options for children with mental illnesses. Disorders affecting children may include anxiety disorders, attention deficit hyperactivity disorder (ADHD), autism spectrum disorders (ASD), bipolar disorder, depression, eating disorders, and schizophrenia.

What Should I Do If I Am Concerned About Mental, Behavioral, Or Emotional Symptoms?

Talk to your doctor or healthcare provider. Ask questions and learn everything you can about the behavior or symptoms that worry you. In the case of children ask the child's teacher if the child has been showing worrisome changes in behavior. Share this with the child's doctor or healthcare provider. Keep in mind that every child is different. Even normal development, such as when children develop language, motor, and social skills, varies from child to child. Ask

About This Chapter: This chapter includes text excerpted from "Treatment Of Children With Mental Illness," National Institute of Mental Health (NIMH), 2009. Reviewed July 2017.

if the child needs further evaluation by a specialist with experience in child behavioral problems. Specialists may include psychiatrists, psychologists, social workers, psychiatric nurses, and behavioral therapists. Educators may also help evaluate children.

How Do I Know If My Problems Are Serious?

Not every problem is serious. In fact, many everyday stresses can cause changes in your behavior. It is important to be able to tell the difference between typical behavior changes and those associated with more serious problems. Pay special attention to behaviors that include:

- Problems across a variety of settings, such as at school, at home, or with peers

- Changes in appetite or sleep

- Social withdrawal, or fearful behavior toward things a child normally is not afraid of

- Returning to behaviors more common in younger children, such as bed-wetting, for a long time

- Signs of being upset, such as sadness or tearfulness

- Signs of self-destructive behavior, such as head-banging, or a tendency to get hurt often

- Repeated thoughts of death

Can Symptoms Be Caused By A Death In The Family, Illness In A Parent, Family Financial Problems, Divorce, Or Other Events?

Yes. Every member of a family is affected by tragedy or extreme stress, even the youngest child. If it takes more than one month for a child to get used to a situation, or if the child has severe reactions, talk to your doctor. Check the child's response to stress. Take note if he or she gets better with time or if professional care is needed. Stressful events are challenging, but they give you a chance to teach the child important ways to cope.

How Are Mental Illnesses Diagnosed?

Before diagnosing a mental illness, the doctor or specialist tries to rule out other possible causes for your behavior. The doctor will:

- Take a history of any important medical problems

- Take a history of the problem—how long you have seen the problem—as well as a history of the child's development

- Take a family history of mental disorders

Survey Finds More Evidence That Mental Disorders Often Begin In Youth

A study using data from the National Institute of Mental Health (NIMH)-funded National Comorbidity Survey-Adolescent Supplement (NCS-A) found that about 20 percent of youth are affected by a mental disorder sometime in their lifetime. The NCS-A is a nationally representative, face-to-face survey of more than 10,000 teens ages 13 to 18. Parents or caregivers were also asked to complete a corroborating questionnaire after teens were interviewed. The NCS-A used criteria established by the American Psychiatric Association's *Diagnostic and Statistical Manual* (DSM-IV) to assess for a wide range of mental disorders including mood and anxiety disorders, behavior disorders like attention deficit hyperactivity disorder (ADHD), eating disorders, and substance use disorders.

In this most recent analysis, Kathleen Merikangas, Ph.D., of NIMH, Ron Kessler, Ph.D., of Harvard University, and colleagues examined the prevalence of mental disorders, as well as the severity of the disorders, within a 12-month period to estimate the rate of serious emotional disturbances (SED) in youth. SED was defined by the Substance Abuse and Mental Health Administration (SAMHSA) as a "mental, behavioral, or emotional disorder… that resulted in functional impairment which substantially interferes with or limits the child's role or functioning in family, school, or community activities."

Results Of The Study

The researchers found that about 8 percent of all respondents had SED. Those with behavior disorders were most likely to be considered to have a severe disorder. Those with three or more coexisting disorders were also more likely to be severely affected. Similar to adults, anxiety disorders were the most common conditions in adolescents. Echoing many other studies, girls were more likely to have a mood or anxiety disorder or eating disorder, while boys were more likely to have a behavior disorder like ADHD or substance use disorder. Contrary to regional studies, this report showed a lower rate of depression among Hispanics compared to whites.

Significance

The findings in the study reflect the widely held belief that most psychiatric disorders first manifest in childhood or adolescence and tend to persist or recur throughout a person's life. The researchers conclude that the high prevalence rate of mental disorders in U.S. adolescents underscores the need for more research focused on changing the trajectory of mental disorders in youth.

(Source: "Survey Finds More Evidence That Mental Disorders Often Begin In Youth," National Institute of Mental Health (NIMH).)

- Ask if the child has experienced physical or psychological traumas, such as a natural disaster, or situations that may cause stress, such as a death in the family

- Consider reports from parents and other caretakers or teachers.

Will I Get Better With Time?

Some adolescents get better with time. But other adolescents need ongoing professional help. Talk to your doctor or specialist about problems that are severe, continuous, and affect daily activities. Also, don't delay seeking help. Treatment may produce better results if started early.

Chapter 48

Treatment Of Children With Mental Illness

Research shows that half of all lifetime cases of mental illness begin by age 14. Scientists are discovering that changes in the body leading to mental illness may start much earlier, before any symptoms appear.

This chapter addresses common questions about treatment options for children with mental illnesses. Disorders affecting children may include anxiety disorders, attention deficit hyperactivity disorder (ADHD), autism spectrum disorders (ASD), bipolar disorder, depression, eating disorders, and schizophrenia.

Treatment Options

In the United States, 75 to 80 percent of children and youth in need of mental health services do not receive them. This can be for a variety of reasons, including

- discrimination and negative attitudes attached to seeking help for mental health issues,
- cultural beliefs and practices,
- access to services/supports,
- availability of providers,
- not knowing where to start, or
- confusion about who to see and what advice to take.

About This Chapter: This chapter includes text excerpted from "Treatment Of Children With Mental Illness: Frequently Asked Questions," National Institute of Mental Health (NIMH), 2014.

> **Treatment Approaches**
>
> Mental health treatment can includes a variety of different approaches and occur in a variety of settings. Services provided depend on the needs and choices of the youth and his or her family, and the diagnosis and severity of the problem. They may consist of services such as psychotherapy with an evidence-based practice, peer mentoring, care coordination, medication, or a combination of all approaches.
>
> *(Source: "Treatment Options," Youth.gov.)*

Are There Treatment Options For Children?

Yes. Once a diagnosis is made, a child specialist will recommend a specific treatment. It is important to understand the various treatment choices, which often include psychotherapy or medication. Talk about the options with a healthcare professional who has experience treating the illness observed in the child. Some treatment choices have been studied experimentally, and other treatments are a part of healthcare practice. In addition, not every community has every type of service or program.

What Are Psychotropic Medications?

Psychotropic medications are substances that affect brain chemicals related to mood and behavior. In recent years, research has been conducted to understand the benefits and risks of using psychotropics in children. Still, more needs to be learned about the effects of psychotropics, especially in children under six years of age. While researchers are trying to clarify how early treatment affects a growing body, families and doctors should weigh the benefits and risks of medication. Each child has individual needs, and each child needs to be monitored closely while taking medications.

Are There Treatments Other Than Medications?

Yes. Psychosocial therapies can be very effective alone and in combination with medications. Psychosocial therapies are also called "talk therapies" or "behavioral therapy," and they help people with mental illness change behavior. Therapies that teach parents and children coping strategies can also be effective.

Cognitive behavioral therapy (CBT) is a type of psychotherapy that can be used with children. It has been widely studied and is an effective treatment for a number of conditions, such as depression, obsessive-compulsive disorder, and social anxiety. A person in CBT learns to change distorted thinking patterns and unhealthy behavior. Children can receive CBT with or without their parents, as well as in a group setting. CBT can be adapted to fit the needs of each child. It is especially useful when treating anxiety disorders.

Additionally, a number of therapies exist for ADHD, oppositional defiant disorder, and conduct disorder and include behavioral parent management training (PMT) and behavioral classroom management. Some children benefit from a combination of different psychosocial approaches. An example is behavioral parent management training in combination with CBT for the child. In other cases, a combination of medication and psychosocial therapies may be most effective. Psychosocial therapies often take time, effort, and patience. However, sometimes children learn new skills that may have positive long-term benefits.

When Is It A Good Idea To Use Psychotropic Medications In Young Children?

When the benefits of treatment outweigh the risks, psychotropic medications may be prescribed. Some children need medication to manage severe and difficult problems. Without treatment, these children would suffer serious or dangerous consequences. In addition, psychosocial treatments may not always be effective by themselves. In some instances, however, they can be quite effective when combined with medication.

For some conditions, the child might be more likely to require medication (e.g., schizophrenia, bipolar disorder), but for many other conditions there are research-supported alternatives to medication (e.g., CBT for anxiety, behavioral PMT for conduct-related problems).

Ask your doctor questions about alternatives to medications and about the risks of starting and continuing on these medications. Learn everything you can about the medications prescribed for the child. Learn about possible side effects, some of which may be harmful. Know what a particular treatment is supposed to do. For example, will it change a specific behavior? If you do not see these changes while the child is taking the medication, talk to his or her doctor. Also, discuss the risks of stopping medication with your doctor.

Does Medication Affect Young Children Differently Than Older Children Or Adults?

Yes. Young children handle medications differently than older children and adults. The brains of young children change and develop rapidly. Studies have found that developing brains can be very sensitive to medications. There are also developmental differences in how children metabolize—how their bodies process—medications. Therefore, doctors should carefully consider the dosage or how much medication to give each child. Much more research is needed to determine the effects and benefits of medications in children of all ages. But keep in mind that serious untreated mental disorders themselves can harm brain development.

Also, it is important to avoid drug interactions. If the child takes medicine for asthma or cold symptoms, talk to your doctor or pharmacist. Drug interactions could cause medications to not work as intended or lead to serious side effects.

How Should Medication Be Included In An Overall Treatment Plan?

Medication should be used with other treatments. It should not be the only treatment. Consider other services, such as family therapy, family support services, educational classes, and behavior management techniques. If the child's doctor prescribes medication, he or she should evaluate the child regularly to make sure the medication is working. Children need treatment plans tailored to their individual problems and needs.

What Medications Are Used For Which Kinds Of Childhood Mental Disorders?

Psychotropic medications include stimulants, antidepressants, antianxiety medications, antipsychotics, and mood stabilizers. Dosages approved by the U.S. Food and Drug Administration (FDA) for use in children depend on body weight and age.

What Does It Mean If A Medication Is Specifically Approved For Use In Children?

When the FDA approves a medication, it means the drug manufacturer provided the agency with information showing the medication is safe and effective in a particular group of people. Based on this information, the drug's label lists proper dosage, potential side effects, and approved age. Medications approved for children follow these guidelines.

Many psychotropic medications have not been studied in children, which means they have not been approved by the FDA for use in children. But doctors may prescribe medications as they feel appropriate, even if those uses are not included on the label. This is called "off-label" use. Research shows that off-label use of some medications works well in some children. Other medications need more study in children. In particular, the use of most psychotropic medications has not been adequately studied in preschoolers.

More studies in children are needed before we can fully know the appropriate dosages, how a medication works in children, and what effects a medication might have on learning and development.

Why Haven't Many Medications Been Tested In Children?

In the past, medications were seldom studied in children because mental illness was not recognized in childhood. Also, there were ethical concerns about involving children in research. This led to a lack of knowledge about the best treatments for children. In clinical settings today, children with mental or behavioral disorders are being prescribed medications at increasingly early ages. The FDA has been urging that medications be appropriately studied in children, and Congress passed legislation in 1997 offering incentives to drug manufacturers to carry out such testing. These activities have helped increase research on the effects of medications in children. There still are ethical concerns about testing medications in children. However, strict rules protect participants in research studies. Each study must go through many types of review before, and after it begins.

What Else Can I Do To Help My Child?

Children with mental illness need guidance and understanding from their parents and teachers. This support can help the child achieve his or her full potential and succeed in school. Before the child is diagnosed, frustration, blame, and anger may have built up within a family. Parents and children may need special help to undo these unhealthy interaction patterns. Mental health professionals can counsel the child and family to help everyone develop new skills, attitudes, and ways of relating to each other.

Parents can also help by taking part in parenting skills training. This helps parents learn how to handle difficult situations and behaviors. Training encourages parents to share a pleasant or relaxing activity with their child, to notice and point out what their child does well, and to praise their child's strengths and abilities. Parents may also learn to arrange family situations in more positive ways. Also, parents may benefit from learning stress-management techniques to help them deal with frustration and respond calmly to their child's behavior.

Sometimes, the whole family may need counseling. Therapists can help family members find better ways to handle disruptive behaviors and encourage behavior changes. Finally, support groups help parents and families connect with others who have similar problems and concerns. Groups often meet regularly to share frustrations and successes, to exchange information about recommended specialists and strategies, and to talk with experts.

Where Can I Go For Help?

If you are unsure where to go for help, ask your family doctor. Others who can help are:

- Mental health specialists, such as psychiatrists, psychologists, social workers, or mental health counselors

- Health maintenance organizations

- Community mental health centers

- Hospital psychiatry departments and outpatient clinics

- Mental health programs at universities or medical schools

- State hospital outpatient clinics

- Family services, social agencies, or clergy

- Peer support groups

- Private clinics and facilities

- Employee assistance programs

- Local medical and/or psychiatric societies.

You can also check the phone book under "mental health," "health," "social services," "hotlines," or "physicians" for phone numbers and addresses. An emergency room doctor can also provide temporary help and can tell you where and how to get further help.

Chapter 49

Finding A Therapist Who Can Help You Heal

Psychotherapy (sometimes called "talk therapy") is a term for a variety of treatment techniques that aim to help a person identify and change troubling emotions, thoughts, and behavior. Most psychotherapy takes place with a licensed and trained mental healthcare professional and a patient meeting one on one or with other patients in a group setting.

Someone might seek out psychotherapy for different reasons:

- You might be dealing with severe or long-term stress from a job or family situation, the loss of a loved one, or relationship or other family issues. Or you may have symptoms with no physical explanation: changes in sleep or appetite, low energy, a lack of interest or pleasure in activities that you once enjoyed, persistent irritability, or a sense of discouragement or hopelessness that won't go away.

- A health professional may suspect or have diagnosed a condition such as depression, bipolar disorder, posttraumatic stress or other disorder and recommended psychotherapy as a first treatment or to go along with medication.

- You may be seeking treatment for a family member or child who has been diagnosed with a condition affecting mental health and for whom a health professional has recommended treatment.

An exam by your primary care practitioner can ensure there is nothing in your overall health that would explain your or a loved one's symptoms.

About This Chapter: Text in this chapter begins with excerpts from "Psychotherapies," National Institute of Mental Health (NIMH), November 2016; Text beginning with the heading "Finding The Right Therapist" is excerpted from "Selecting And Working With A Therapist Skilled In Adoption," Child Welfare Information Gateway, U.S. Department of Health and Human Services (HHS), July 2012. Reviewed July 2017.

Several types of psychotherapy or "talk therapy" can help people with depression. Some treatments are short-term, lasting 10 to 20 weeks, and others are longer, depending on the person's needs.

- Cognitive Behavioral Therapy (CBT)
- Interpersonal Therapy (IPT)
- Problem-Solving Therapy (PST)

(Source: "Depression: Psychotherapy," NIHSeniorHealth, National Institute on Aging (NIA).)

What To Consider When Looking For A Therapist

Therapists have different professional backgrounds and specialties. There are resources at the end of this chapter that can help you find out about the different credentials of therapists and resources for locating therapists.

There are many different types of psychotherapy. Different therapies are often variations on an established approach, such as cognitive behavioral therapy. There is no formal approval process for psychotherapies as there is for the use of medications in medicine. For many therapies, however, research involving large numbers of patients has provided evidence that treatment is effective for specific disorders. These "evidence-based therapies" have been shown in research to reduce symptoms of depression, anxiety, and other disorders.

The particular approach a therapist uses depends on the condition being treated and the training and experience of the therapist. Also, therapists may combine and adapt elements of different approaches.

One goal of establishing an evidence base for psychotherapies is to prevent situations in which a person receives therapy for months or years with no benefit. If you have been in therapy and feel you are not getting better, talk to your therapist, or look into other practitioners or approaches. The object of therapy is to gain relief from symptoms and improve quality of life.

Once you have identified one or more possible therapists, a preliminary conversation with a therapist can help you get an idea of how treatment will proceed and whether you feel comfortable with the therapist. Rapport and trust are important. Discussions in therapy are deeply personal and it's important that you feel comfortable and trusting with the therapist and have confidence in his or her expertise.

Consider asking the following questions:

- What are the credentials and experience of the therapist? Does he or she have a specialty?

- What approach will the therapist take to help you? Does he or she practice a particular type of therapy? What can the therapist tell you about the rationale for the therapy and the evidence base?

- Does the therapist have experience in diagnosing and treating the age group (for example, a child) and the specific condition for which treatment is being sought? If a child is the patient, how will parents be involved in treatment?

- What are the goals of therapy? Does the therapist recommend a specific time frame or number of sessions? How will progress be assessed and what happens if you (or the therapist) feel you aren't starting to feel better?

- Will there be homework?

- Are medications an option? How will medications be prescribed if the therapist is not an M.D.?

- Are our meetings confidential? How can this be assured?

Elements Of Psychotherapy

A variety of different kinds of psychotherapies and interventions have been shown to be effective for specific disorders. Psychotherapists may use one primary approach, or incorporate different elements depending on their training, the condition being treated, and the needs of the person receiving treatment.

Here are examples of the elements that psychotherapies can include:

- Helping a person become aware of ways of thinking that may be automatic but are inaccurate and harmful. (An example might be someone who has a low opinion of his or her own abilities). The therapist helps the person find ways to question these thoughts, understand how they affect emotions and behavior, and try ways to change self-defeating patterns. This approach is central to cognitive behavioral therapy (CBT).

- Identifying ways to cope with stress.

- Examining in depth a person's interactions with others and offering guidance with social and communication skills, if needed.

- Relaxation and mindfulness techniques.

- Exposure therapy for people with anxiety disorders. In exposure therapy, a person spends brief periods, in a supportive environment, learning to tolerate the distress certain items, ideas, or imagined scenes cause. Over time the fear associated with these things dissipates.

- Tracking emotions and activities and the impact of each on the other.

- Safety planning can include helping a person recognize warning signs, and thinking about coping strategies, such as contacting friends, family, or emergency personnel.

- Supportive counseling to help a person explore troubling issues and provide emotional support.

eHealth

The telephone, Internet, and mobile devices have opened up new possibilities for providing interventions that can reach people in areas where mental health professionals may be not be easily available, and can be at hand 24/7. Some of these approaches involve a therapist providing help at a distance, but others—such as web-based programs and cell phone apps—are designed to provide information and feedback in the absence of a therapist. Some approaches that use electronic media to provide help for mental health-related conditions have been shown by research to be helpful in some situations, others not as yet.

Taking The First Step

The symptoms of mental disorders can have a profound effect on someone's quality of life and ability to function. Treatment can address symptoms as well as assist someone experiencing severe or ongoing stress. Some of the reasons that you might consider seeking out psychotherapy include:

- Overwhelming sadness or helplessness that doesn't go away

- Serious, unusual insomnia, or sleeping too much

- Difficulty focusing on work, or carrying out other everyday activities

- Constant worry and anxiety

- Drinking to excess or any behavior that harms self or others

- Dealing with a difficult transition, such as a divorce, children leaving home, job difficulties, or the death of someone close

- Children's behavior problems that interfere with school, family, or peers

Seeking help is not an admission of weakness, but a step towards understanding and obtaining relief from distressing symptoms.

Finding The Right Therapist

Locating the right therapist requires that we identify some prospective therapists who have adoption experience and then conduct preliminary interviews to find the one who seems best able to help the child or family.

Identifying prospective therapists. It is important that we take the time to find a mental health provider who has the experience and expertise required to address their needs effectively. Because adopted children can present the same problems common to all children, the therapist must first be a skilled diagnostician in order to determine what is an adoption problem and what is not. Professionals with adoption, attachment, and trauma knowledge and experience are best suited to help families determine whether problems are adoption-related and to plan effective treatment strategies. At a minimum, a therapist must:

- Be knowledgeable about adoption and the psychological impact of adoption on children and families

- Be knowledgeable about the impact of trauma on children and families, as the most serious problems result from traumatic experiences prior to adoption

- Be knowledgeable about the role and impact of attachment on the mind/body for the developing child

- Be experienced in working with adopted children and their families

- Know the types of help available for adoption-related issues and problems

- Have received training in working with adoptive families

We may contact community adoption support networks, ask their placement agency for referrals to therapists, or search online. Many public and private adoption agencies and adoptive parent support groups have lists of therapists who have been trained in adoption issues or who have effectively worked with children in foster care and adoption. Some adoption agencies and specialized postadoption service agencies have mental health therapists trained in adoption on staff.

We can check with the following resources for therapist recommendations:

- Agency social workers involved in the child's adoption

- State or local mental health associations

- Public and private adoption agencies

- Local adoptive parent support groups

- Specialized postadoption service agencies

- State adoption offices

- National and State professional organizations (see National Resource Organizations)

Interviewing prospective therapists. Using the recommendations that they gather, we can call prospective therapists or schedule an initial interview to find out basic information. Some therapists will offer an initial brief consultation that is free of charge. We should start by giving the clinician a brief description of the concern or problem for which they need help. Some questions to discuss follow:

- What is your experience with adoption and adoption issues? (Parents should be specific about the adoption issues that affect their problem, such as open adoption, transracial adoption, searching for birth relatives, children who have experienced abuse or institutionalization, or children with attachment difficulties.)

- How long have you been in practice, and what degrees, licenses, or certifications do you have?

- What continuing clinical training have you had on adoption issues?

- Who oversaw your training?

- Do you include parents and other family members in the therapeutic process?

- Do you prefer to work with the entire family or only with the children?

- Do you give parents regular reports on a child's progress?

- Can you estimate a timeframe for the course of therapy?

- What approach to therapy do you use?

- What changes in the daily life of the child and family might we expect to see as a result of the therapy?

- Do you work with teachers, juvenile justice personnel, daycare providers, and other adults in the child's life, when appropriate?

There are other practical considerations when choosing a therapist. We should be sure to ask about:

- Coverage when the therapist is not available, especially in an emergency

- Appointment times and availability

- Fees and whether the therapist accepts specific insurance, adoption subsidy medical payments, or Medicaid reimbursement payments (if applicable)

Working With A Therapist

If the child is the identified client in therapy, the family's involvement and support for the therapy is critical to a positive outcome for him or her. An adoption-competent therapist will value the participation of adoptive parents. Traditional family therapists who are unfamiliar with adoption issues may view the child's problems as a manifestation of overall family dysfunction. They may not take into account the child's earlier experiences in other care settings and may view adoptive parents more as a part of the problem than the solution. Adoption competent therapists know that the adoptive parents will be empowered by including them in the therapeutic process and that no intervention should threaten the parent-child relationship.

Parents' commitment to the therapy may also contribute to the success of the therapeutic process. For instance, parents are obligated to keep scheduled appointments. They should refrain from using therapy sessions as punishment for a child's misbehavior. Family members must communicate regularly with the therapist and ensure that the therapist has regular feedback about conditions at home. The success of therapy depends heavily on open and trusting communication.

We may want to request an evaluation meeting with the therapist 6 to 8 weeks after treatment begins and regular updates thereafter. Evaluation meetings will help all parties evaluate the progress of treatment and offer the opportunity to discuss the following:

- Satisfaction with the working relationship between the therapist and family members

- Progress toward mutually agreed-on goals for treatment approaches and desired outcomes

- Progress on problems that first prompted the request for treatment

- The therapist's tentative diagnosis (usually necessary for insurance reimbursement)

- The therapist's evaluation of whether therapy can improve the situation that prompted treatment

Even when the match with a therapist appears to be perfect, the relationship with the family or the results may not be satisfactory. We must be willing to change therapists when the therapy does not appear to be progressing appropriately. Parents are the experts about their own children and are the ones who must decide what makes sense for their children. It is worthwhile to discuss a move with the therapist, but the parents are the ones responsible for arranging effective treatment.

Chapter 50

Going To Therapy: What To Expect

Lots of teens have some kind of emotional problem. In fact, almost half of U.S. teens will have a mental health problem before they turn 18. The good news is that therapy can really help. Sometimes, people are embarrassed or afraid to see a therapist. But getting help from a therapist because you're feeling sad or anxious is really not different from seeing a doctor because you broke a bone. In fact, you can feel proud for being brave enough to do what you need to do to get your life back on track.

What Is Therapy?

Therapy is when you talk about your problems with someone who is a professional counselor, such as a psychiatrist, psychologist, or social worker. Therapy sometimes is called psychotherapy. That is because it helps with your psychology—the mental and emotional parts of your life.

If you are going through a rough time, talking to a caring therapist can be a great relief. A therapist can help you cope with sadness, worry, and other strong or scary feelings. Here are some other ways therapy can help:

- It can teach you specific skills for handling difficult situations, such as problems with your family or school.

- It can help you find healthy ways to deal with stress or anger.

- It can teach you how to build healthy relationships.

About This Chapter: This chapter includes text excerpted from "Going To Therapy," girlshealth.gov, Office on Women's Health (OWH), January 7, 2015.

- It can help you figure out how to think about things in more positive ways.

- It can help you figure out how to boost your self-confidence.

- It can help you decide where you want to go in life and how to deal with any obstacles that may come up along the way.

Therapy may feel great right away, or it might feel strange at first. It can take a little time getting used to talking with someone new about your problems. But therapists are trained to listen well, and they want to help. As time goes on, you should feel comfortable with your therapist. If you don't feel comfortable, or if you think you're not getting better, tell your parent or guardian. Another therapist or type of therapy might work better.

Therapists protect people's privacy. They can share what you say only in very special cases, such as if they think you are in danger. If you're concerned, though, ask about the privacy policy. It's important to feel like you can tell the truth in therapy. It works best if you are honest about any problems you're facing, including problems with drugs or alcohol or any behaviors that can hurt your body or mind.

Just because you start to see a therapist doesn't mean that you will see one forever. You should be able to learn skills that let you handle your problems on your own. Sometimes, a few sessions are all you need to learn skills and feel better.

Why Do Teens Go For Therapy?

Many young people develop mental health conditions, like depression, eating disorders, or anxiety disorders. If you have a mental health problem, remember there are treatments that work, and you can feel better.

Also, some teens go to therapy to get help through a tough time, like their parents' getting divorced or having too much stress at school. If you feel out of control, or you feel like a mental health problem keeps you from enjoying life, get help. Reach out to a parent or guardian or another trusted adult.

What Should I Do To Get Started With Therapy?

If you need help finding a therapist, you can start by talking to your doctor, school nurse, or school counselor. If your family has insurance, the insurance company can tell you which therapists are covered under your plan. You and your parent or guardian also can look online for mental health treatment on this webpage (findtreatment.samhsa.gov/locator/home).

If you need help paying for therapy, you can ask a parent or guardian if they have health insurance that might help pay for therapy. If your family doesn't have insurance, they can find out about getting it through healthcare.gov. You also may be able to get free or low-cost therapy at a mental health clinic, hospital, university, or other places.

What Are Some Kinds Of Therapy?

There are different kinds of therapy to help you feel better. The best treatment depends on the type of problem that you are facing.

You may have one-on-one talk therapy. This is when you talk to a therapist alone. Or you may join group therapy, where you work with a therapist and other people who are having similar issues. You may also do art therapy, where you paint or draw. One kind of talk therapy that tends to work well for depression, anxiety, and several other problems is cognitive behavioral therapy. This type of therapy teaches you how to think and act in healthier ways.

Sometimes, your therapist will suggest that you take medicine in addition to therapy, which often can be a helpful combination.

What About Online Support Groups?

There are lots of support groups available on the Internet, including ones to help you handle your feelings. Chat rooms and other online options may help you feel less alone. But if you are having trouble coping, it's important to work with a therapist or other mental health professional.

Remember to be careful about getting info online. Some people use the Internet to promote unhealthy behaviors, like cutting and dangerous eating habits.

Benefits For Young People

Mentoring is often one component of support programs that involves other elements, such as tutoring or life skills training and coaching. The supportive, healthy relationships formed between mentors and mentees are both immediate and long-term and contribute to a host of benefits for mentors and mentees.

Benefits for youth:

- Increased high school graduation rates
- Lower high school dropout rates

- Healthier relationships and lifestyle choices
- Better attitude about school
- Higher college enrollment rates and higher educational aspirations
- Enhanced self-esteem and self-confidence
- Improved behavior, both at home and at school
- Stronger relationships with parents, teachers, and peers
- Improved interpersonal skills
- Decreased likelihood of initiating drug and alcohol use

(Source: "Benefits For Young People," Youth.gov.)

Chapter 51

Counseling And Therapy: Methods Of Treatment

Cognitive Behavioral Therapy (CBT)

Cognitive behavioral therapy (CBT) is a well established treatment for people with depression. CBT is a blend of two therapies: cognitive therapy and behavioral therapy. Cognitive therapy focuses on a person's thoughts and beliefs, and how they influence a person's mood and actions, and aims to change a person's thinking to be more adaptive and healthy. Behavioral therapy focuses on a person's actions and aims to change unhealthy behavior patterns. CBT helps a person focus on his or her current problems and how to solve them. Both patient and therapist need to be actively involved in this process. The therapist helps the patient learn how to identify and correct distorted thoughts or negative self-talk often associated with depressed feelings, recognize and change inaccurate beliefs, engage in more enjoyable activities, relate to self and others in more positive ways, learn problem-solving skills, and change behaviors. another focus of CBT is behavioral activation (i.e., increasing activity levels and helping the patient take part in rewarding activities which can improve mood). CBT is a structured, weekly intervention. Weekly homework assignments help the individual apply the learned techniques.

About This Chapter: Text beginning with the heading "Cognitive Behavioral Therapy (CBT)" is excerpted from "What Is Major Depression?" U.S. Department of Veterans Affairs (VA), December 2015; Text under the heading "Interpersonal Psychotherapy (IPT)" is excerpted from "Mental Health—Interpersonal Psychotherapy (IPT)," U.S. Department of Veterans Affairs (VA), December 9, 2015; Text under the heading "Dialectical Behavior Therapy (DBT)" is excerpted from "Mental Health Information—Borderline Personality Disorder," National Institute of Mental Health (NIMH), August 2016; Text under the heading "Getting Help Through Therapy" is excerpted from "Mental Health Conditions," girlshealth.gov, Office on Women's Health (OWH), February 16, 2011. Reviewed July 2017.

Cognitive-Behavioral Therapy (CBT) was developed as a method to prevent relapse when treating problem drinking, and later it was adapted for cocaine-addicted individuals. Cognitive-behavioral strategies are based on the theory that in the development of maladaptive behavioral patterns like substance abuse, learning processes play a critical role. Individuals in CBT learn to identify and correct problematic behaviors by applying a range of different skills that can be used to stop drug abuse and to address a range of other problems that often cooccur with it.

A central element of CBT is anticipating likely problems and enhancing patients' self-control by helping them develop effective coping strategies. Specific techniques include exploring the positive and negative consequences of continued drug use, self-monitoring to recognize cravings early and identify situations that might put one at risk for use, and developing strategies for coping with cravings and avoiding those high-risk situations. Research indicates that the skills individuals learn through cognitive-behavioral approaches remain after the completion of treatment.

(Source: "Cognitive-Behavioral Therapy (Alcohol, Marijuana, Cocaine, Methamphetamine, Nicotine)," National Institute on Drug Abuse (NIDA).)

Family Psychoeducation

Mental illness affects the whole family. Family treatment can play an important role to help both the person with depression and his or her relatives. Family psychoeducation is one way families can work together towards recovery. The family and clinician will meet together to discuss the problems they are experiencing. Families will then attend educational sessions where they will learn basic facts about mental illness, coping skills, communication skills, problem-solving skills, and ways to work together toward recovery.

Interpersonal Psychotherapy (IPT)

Interpersonal psychotherapy (IPT) is a treatment for depression that focuses on relationship issues that may be the cause or the result of depression. Many studies have been done that support the usefulness of IPT for depression. Also, studies have shown IPT to be useful in the treatment of other issues such as anxiety, bipolar disorder, eating disorders, and borderline personality disorder.

IPT is typically delivered during 16 weekly sessions over three phases of treatment (Initial Sessions, Intermediate Sessions, and Termination). During the Initial Sessions, the therapist will provide you with education about depression, how your life situations may be contributing to depression, and how depression may affect your daily life. The Intermediate Sessions focus on one or two problem areas that are most concerning to you and may be contributing to your depression. These areas include dealing with major life changes, conflict with others, grief related to the death of a significant person, or problems making or keeping social connections. During Termination, the therapist will work with you to review progress, explore possible stressors that may contribute to depression, discuss how skills learned in IPT can continue to be used, and evaluate the need for further treatment.

Goals are established early in treatment. One of the most important factors in the success of therapy is a commitment to participating in treatment and regularly attending sessions. In IPT, you would typically meet one-on-one with your therapist for 12–16 sessions. Sessions are generally held on a weekly basis and last approximately 50 minutes. The information you learn during the therapy sessions will be important to you as you apply it to everyday life in order to feel better.

If you decide to participate in IPT, you will be asked to:

- Attend sessions regularly
- Work with your therapist to set therapy goals
- Discuss relationship issues during each session
- Practice new skills—both in and outside of session

Dialectical Behavior Therapy (DBT)

This type of therapy utilizes the concept of mindfulness, or being aware of and attentive to the current situation and moods. Dialectical behavior therapy (DBT) also teaches skills to control intense emotions, reduce self-destructive behaviors, and improve relationships. DBT differs from CBT in that it integrates traditional CBT elements with mindfulness, acceptance, and techniques to improve a person's ability to tolerate stress and control his or her emotions. DBT recognizes the dialectical tension between the need for acceptance and the need for change.

Getting Help Through Therapy

Your treatment probably will include some sessions of therapy. That means talking to a professional counselor like a psychologist, psychiatrist, or social worker. If you feel uncomfortable about needing therapy, remember that getting help for your brain isn't very different from getting help for your stomach, teeth, or any other part of you.

Of course, it can take a little time getting used to talking with someone about your problems. But therapists are trained to listen well, and they want to help. Also, therapists care a lot about protecting people's privacy. If you're concerned, though, ask about the privacy policy. As time goes on, you should feel comfortable with your therapist. If you don't, or if you think you're not getting better, tell your parent or guardian.

Lots of people feel relief just from sharing their feelings and getting emotional support. That's certainly part of therapy. But therapy also can teach you specific skills for coping with problems. It also can help you find ways to deal with stress and build healthy relationships. And it can help you figure out where you want to go in life and how to deal with any obstacles to getting there.

There are different types of therapy, and the kind you have can depend on the problems you're facing. One kind of therapy that tends to work well for depression, social anxiety, and several other problems is cognitive behavioral therapy, which teaches you ways to make your thoughts and behaviors healthier.

You also might go to group therapy. At group therapy, you will work with a therapist and other people who have problems like yours. There's also play and art therapy, where you work on your feelings through playing or drawing and other creative activities. Therapy also could be with your family.

There are several other types of therapy as well. Whatever form it takes, therapy works best if you're honest about any problems you're facing at school or at home—or with drugs, alcohol, or any behaviors that can hurt your body and your mind.

Chapter 52

Common Mental Health Medications

Medications can play a role in treating several mental disorders and conditions. Treatment may also include psychotherapy (also called "talk therapy") and brain stimulation therapies (less common). In some cases, psychotherapy alone may be the best treatment option. Choosing the right treatment plan should be based on a person's individual needs and medical situation, and under a mental health professional's care.

Information about medications changes frequently. Check the U.S. Food and Drug Administration (FDA) website (www.fda.gov) for the latest warnings, patient medication guides, or newly approved medications. You can search by brand name on MedlinePlus Drugs, Herbs, and Supplements Drugs website (www.medlineplus.gov). The MedlinePlus website also provides additional information about each medication, including side effects and FDA warnings.

> Prescription medications also are an important resource for treating mental disorders. Medications for mental disorders provide significant relief for many people and help manage symptoms to the point where people can use other strategies to pursue recovery. Medications work better for some people than others, even if they have the same disorders.
>
> Medication effectiveness can also change over time, so it is not uncommon for a person to find that the medication needs to be changed or adjusted even after it has been working. Medications also often have significant side effects. As a result, it is important for people receiving medications for behavioral health problems to have regular contact with the prescribing provider to ensure that the approach being used continues to be safe and effective.

About This Chapter: This chapter includes text excerpted from "Mental Health Medications," National Institute of Mental Health (NIMH), October 2016.

> Medication tends to be most effective when it is used in combination with counseling or psychotherapy. There are many different types of medication for mental health problems, including anti-depressants, medication for attention issues, anti-anxiety medications, mood stabilizers, and antipsychotic medications.
>
> *(Source: "Behavioral Health Treatments And Services," Substance Abuse and Mental Health Services Administration (SAMHSA).)*

Understanding Your Medications

If you are prescribed a medication, be sure that you:

- Tell the doctor about all medications and vitamin supplements you are already taking.

- Remind your doctor about any allergies and any problems you have had with medicines.

- Understand how to take the medicine before you start using it and take your medicine as instructed.

- Don't take medicines prescribed for another person or give yours to someone else.

- Call your doctor right away if you have any problems with your medicine or if you are worried that it might be doing more harm than good. Your doctor may be able to adjust the dose or change your prescription to a different one that may work better for you.

Antidepressants

What Are Antidepressants?

Antidepressants are medications commonly used to treat depression. Antidepressants are also used for other health conditions, such as anxiety, pain and insomnia. Although antidepressants are not FDA-approved specifically to treat attention deficit hyperactivity disorder (ADHD), antidepressants are sometimes used to treat ADHD in adults.

The most popular types of antidepressants are called selective serotonin reuptake inhibitors (SSRIs). Examples of SSRIs include:

- Fluoxetine
- Citalopram
- Sertraline
- Paroxetine
- Escitalopram

Other types of antidepressants are serotonin and norepinephrine reuptake inhibitors (SNRIs). SNRIs are similar to SSRIs and include venlafaxine and duloxetine. Another antidepressant that is commonly used is bupropion. Bupropion is a third type of antidepressant which works differently than either SSRIs or SNRIs. Bupropion is also used to treat seasonal affective disorder and to help people stop smoking.

SSRIs, SNRIs, and bupropion are popular because they do not cause as many side effects as older classes of antidepressants, and seem to help a broader group of depressive and anxiety disorders. Older antidepressant medications include tricyclics, tetracyclics, and monoamine oxidase inhibitors (MAOIs). For some people, tricyclics, tetracyclics, or MAOIs may be the best medications.

How Do People Respond To Antidepressants?

According to a research review by the Agency for Healthcare Research and Quality (AHRQ), all antidepressant medications work about as well as each other to improve symptoms of depression and to keep depression symptoms from coming back. For reasons not yet well understood, some people respond better to some antidepressant medications than to others.

Therefore, it is important to know that some people may not feel better with the first medicine they try and may need to try several medicines to find the one that works for them. Others may find that a medicine helped for a while, but their symptoms came back. It is important to carefully follow your doctor's directions for taking your medicine at an adequate dose and over an extended period of time (often 4 to 6 weeks) for it to work.

Once a person begins taking antidepressants, it is important to not stop taking them without the help of a doctor. Sometimes people taking antidepressants feel better and stop taking the medication too soon, and the depression may return. When it is time to stop the medication, the doctor will help the person slowly and safely decrease the dose. It's important to give the body time to adjust to the change. People don't get addicted (or "hooked") on these medications, but stopping them abruptly may also cause withdrawal symptoms.

What Are The Possible Side Effects Of Antidepressants?

Some antidepressants may cause more side effects than others. You may need to try several different antidepressant medications before finding the one that improves your symptoms and that causes side effects that you can manage.

The most common side effects listed by the FDA include:

- Nausea and vomiting
- Weight gain
- Diarrhea
- Sleepiness
- Sexual problems

Call your doctor right away if you have any of the following symptoms, especially if they are new, worsening, or worry you:

- Thoughts about suicide or dying
- Attempts to commit suicide
- New or worsening depression
- New or worsening anxiety
- Feeling very agitated or restless
- Panic attacks
- Trouble sleeping (insomnia)
- New or worsening irritability
- Acting aggressively, being angry, or violent
- Acting on dangerous impulses
- An extreme increase in activity and talking (mania)
- Other unusual changes in behavior or mood

Combining the newer SSRI or SNRI antidepressants with one of the commonly-used "triptan" medications used to treat migraine headaches could cause a life-threatening illness called "serotonin syndrome." A person with serotonin syndrome may be agitated, have hallucinations (see or hear things that are not real), have a high temperature, or have unusual blood pressure changes. Serotonin syndrome is usually associated with the older antidepressants called MAOIs, but it can happen with the newer antidepressants as well, if they are mixed with the wrong medications. Antidepressants may cause other side effects that were not included in this list. To report any serious adverse effects associated with the use of antidepressant medicines, please contact the FDA MedWatch program using the contact information at the bottom of this page.

Antianxiety Medications

What Are Antianxiety Medications?

Antianxiety medications help reduce the symptoms of anxiety, such as panic attacks, or extreme fear and worry. The most common antianxiety medications are called benzodiazepines. Benzodiazepines can treat generalized anxiety disorder. In the case of panic disorder or social phobia (social anxiety disorder), benzodiazepines are usually second-line treatments, behind SSRIs or other antidepressants.

Benzodiazepines used to treat anxiety disorders include:

- Clonazepam

- Alprazolam

- Lorazepam

Short half-life (or short-acting) benzodiazepines (such as Lorazepam) and beta blockers are used to treat the short-term symptoms of anxiety. Beta blockers help manage physical symptoms of anxiety, such as trembling, rapid heartbeat, and sweating that people with phobias (an overwhelming and unreasonable fear of an object or situation, such as public speaking) experience in difficult situations. Taking these medications for a short period of time can help the person keep physical symptoms under control and can be used "as needed" to reduce acute anxiety.

Buspirone (which is unrelated to the benzodiazepines) is sometimes used for the long-term treatment of chronic anxiety. In contrast to the benzodiazepines, buspirone must be taken every day for a few weeks to reach its full effect. It is not useful on an "as-needed" basis.

How Do People Respond To Antianxiety Medications?

Antianxiety medications such as benzodiazepines are effective in relieving anxiety and take effect more quickly than the antidepressant medications (or buspirone) often prescribed for anxiety. However, people can buildup a tolerance to benzodiazepines if they are taken over a long period of time and may need higher and higher doses to get the same effect. Some people may even become dependent on them. To avoid these problems, doctors usually prescribe benzodiazepines for short periods, a practice that is especially helpful for older adults, people who have substance abuse problems and people who become dependent on medication easily. If people suddenly stop taking benzodiazepines, they may have withdrawal symptoms or their anxiety may return. Therefore, benzodiazepines should be tapered off slowly.

What Are The Possible Side Effects Of Antianxiety Medications?

Like other medications, antianxiety medications may cause side effects. Some of these side effects and risks are serious. The most common side effects for benzodiazepines are drowsiness and dizziness. Other possible side effects include:

- Nausea
- Blurred vision
- Headache

- Confusion
- Tiredness
- Nightmares

Tell your doctor if any of these symptoms are severe or do not go away:

- Drowsiness
- Dizziness
- Unsteadiness
- Problems with coordination
- Difficulty thinking or remembering
- Increased saliva
- Muscle or joint pain
- Frequent urination
- Blurred vision
- Changes in sex drive or ability (The American Society of Health-System Pharmacists, Inc, 2010)

If you experience any of the symptoms below, call your doctor immediately:

- Rash
- Hives
- Swelling of the eyes, face, lips, tongue, or throat
- Difficulty breathing or swallowing
- Hoarseness
- Seizures
- Yellowing of the skin or eyes

- Depression

- Difficulty speaking

- Yellowing of the skin or eyes

- Thoughts of suicide or harming yourself

- Difficulty breathing

Common side effects of beta blockers include:

- Fatigue

- Cold hands

- Dizziness or light-headedness

- Weakness

Beta blockers generally are not recommended for people with asthma or diabetes because they may worsen symptoms related to both.

Possible side effects from buspirone include:

- Dizziness

- Headaches

- Nausea

- Nervousness

- Lightheadedness

- Excitement

- Trouble sleeping

Antianxiety medications may cause other side effects that are not included in the lists above.

Stimulants

What Are Stimulants?

As the name suggests, stimulants increase alertness, attention, and energy, as well as elevate blood pressure, heart rate, and respiration (National Institute on Drug Abuse (NIDA), 2014).

Stimulant medications are often prescribed to treat children, adolescents, or adults diagnosed with ADHD.

Stimulants used to treat ADHD include:

- Methylphenidate

- Amphetamine

- Dextroamphetamine

- Lisdexamfetamine Dimesylate

In 2002, the U.S. Food and Drug Administration (FDA) approved the nonstimulant medication atomoxetine for use as a treatment for ADHD. Two other nonstimulant antihypertensive medications, clonidine and guanfacine, are also approved for treatment of ADHD in children and adolescents. One of these nonstimulant medications is often tried first in a young person with ADHD, and if response is insufficient, then a stimulant is prescribed.

Stimulants are also prescribed to treat other health conditions, including narcolepsy, and occasionally depression (especially in older or chronically medically ill people and in those who have not responded to other treatments)

How Do People Respond To Stimulants?

Prescription stimulants have a calming and "focusing" effect on individuals with ADHD. Stimulant medications are safe when given under a doctor's supervision. Some children taking them may feel slightly different or "funny."

Some parents worry that stimulant medications may lead to drug abuse or dependence, but there is little evidence of this when they are used properly as prescribed. Additionally, research shows that teens with ADHD who took stimulant medications were less likely to abuse drugs than those who did not take stimulant medications.

What Are The Possible Side Effects Of Stimulants?

Stimulants may cause side effects. Most side effects are minor and disappear when dosage levels are lowered. The most common side effects include:

- Difficulty falling asleep or staying asleep

- Loss of appetite

- Stomach pain

- Headache

Less common side effects include:

- Motor tics or verbal tics (sudden, repetitive movements or sounds)

- Personality changes, such as appearing "flat" or without emotion

Antipsychotics

What Are Antipsychotics?

Antipsychotic medicines are primarily used to manage psychosis. The word "psychosis" is used to describe conditions that affect the mind, and in which there has been some loss of contact with reality, often including delusions (false, fixed beliefs) or hallucinations (hearing or seeing things that are not really there). It can be a symptom of a physical condition such as drug abuse or a mental disorder such as schizophrenia, bipolar disorder, or very severe depression (also known as "psychotic depression").

Antipsychotic medications are often used in combination with other medications to treat delirium, dementia, and mental health conditions, including:

- Attention deficit hyperactivity disorder (ADHD)

- Severe depression

- Eating disorders

- Posttraumatic stress disorder (PTSD)

- Obsessive-compulsive disorder (OCD)

- Generalized anxiety disorder

Antipsychotic medicines do not cure these conditions. They are used to help relieve symptoms and improve quality of life.

Older or first-generation antipsychotic medications are also called conventional "typical" antipsychotics or "neuroleptics." Some of the common typical antipsychotics include:

- Chlorpromazine

- Haloperidol

- Perphenazine

- Fluphenazine

Newer or second generation medications are also called "atypical" antipsychotics. Some of the common atypical antipsychotics include:

- Risperidone

- Olanzapine

- Quetiapine

- Ziprasidone

- Aripiprazole

- Paliperidone

- Lurasidone

According to a 2013 research review by the Agency for Healthcare Research and Quality (AHRQ), typical and atypical antipsychotics both work to treat symptoms of schizophrenia and the manic phase of bipolar disorder.

Several atypical antipsychotics have a "broader spectrum" of action than the older medications, and are used for treating bipolar depression or depression that has not responded to an antidepressant medication alone.

How Do People Respond To Antipsychotics?

Certain symptoms, such as feeling agitated and having hallucinations, usually go away within days of starting an antipsychotic medication. Symptoms like delusions usually go away within a few weeks, but the full effects of the medication may not be seen for up to six weeks. Every patient responds differently, so it may take several trials of different antipsychotic medications to find the one that works best.

Some people may have a relapse—meaning their symptoms come back or get worse. Usually relapses happen when people stop taking their medication, or when they only take it sometimes. Some people stop taking the medication because they feel better or they may feel that they don't need it anymore, but no one should stop taking an antipsychotic medication without talking to his or her doctor. When a doctor says it is okay to stop taking a medication, it should be gradually tapered off—never stopped suddenly. Many people must stay on an antipsychotic continuously for months or years in order to stay well; treatment should be personalized for each individual.

What Are The Possible Side Effects Of Antipsychotics?

Antipsychotics have many side effects (or adverse events) and risks. The FDA lists the following side effects of antipsychotic medicines:

- Drowsiness

- Dizziness

- Restlessness

- Weight gain (the risk is higher with some atypical antipsychotic medicines)

- Dry mouth

- Constipation

- Nausea

- Vomiting

- Blurred vision

- Low blood pressure

- Uncontrollable movements, such as tics and tremors (the risk is higher with typical antipsychotic medicines)

- Seizures

- A low number of white blood cells, which fight infections

A person taking an atypical antipsychotic medication should have his or her weight, glucose levels, and lipid levels monitored regularly by a doctor.

Typical antipsychotic medications can also cause additional side effects related to physical movement, such as:

- Rigidity

- Persistent muscle spasms

- Tremors

- Restlessness

Long-term use of typical antipsychotic medications may lead to a condition called tardive dyskinesia (TD). TD causes muscle movements, commonly around the mouth, that a person can't control. TD can range from mild to severe, and in some people, the problem cannot be cured. Sometimes people with TD recover partially or fully after they stop taking typical antipsychotic medication. People who think that they might have TD should check with their doctor before stopping their medication. TD rarely occurs while taking atypical antipsychotics.

Antipsychotics may cause other side effects that are not included in this list above. To report any serious adverse effects associated with the use of these medicines, please contact the FDA MedWatch program (www.fda.gov/Safety/MedWatch).

Mood Stabilizers

What Are Mood Stabilizers?

Mood stabilizers are used primarily to treat bipolar disorder, mood swings associated with other mental disorders, and in some cases, to augment the effect of other medications used to treat depression. Lithium, which is an effective mood stabilizer, is approved for the treatment of mania and the maintenance treatment of bipolar disorder. A number of cohort studies describe antisuicide benefits of lithium for individuals on long-term maintenance. Mood stabilizers work by decreasing abnormal activity in the brain and are also sometimes used to treat:

- Depression (usually along with an antidepressant)

- Schizoaffective Disorder

- Disorders of impulse control

- Certain mental illnesses in children

Anticonvulsant medications are also used as mood stabilizers. They were originally developed to treat seizures, but they were found to help control unstable moods as well. One anticonvulsant commonly used as a mood stabilizer is valproic acid (also called divalproex sodium). For some people, especially those with "mixed" symptoms of mania and depression or those with rapid-cycling bipolar disorder, valproic acid may work better than lithium. Other anticonvulsants used as mood stabilizers include:

- Carbamazepine

- Oxcarbazepine

- Lamotrigine

What Are The Possible Side Effects Of Mood Stabilizers?

Mood stabilizers can cause several side effects, and some of them may become serious, especially at excessively high blood levels.

These side effects include:

- Itching, rash

- Excessive thirst

- Frequent urination

- Tremor (shakiness) of the hands

- Nausea and vomiting

- Slurred speech

- Fast, slow, irregular, or pounding heartbeat

- Blackouts

- Changes in vision

- Seizures

- Hallucinations (seeing things or hearing voices that do not exist)

- Loss of coordination

- Swelling of the eyes, face, lips, tongue, throat, hands, feet, ankles, or lower legs.

If a person with bipolar disorder is being treated with lithium, he or she should visit the doctor regularly to check the lithium levels his or her blood, and make sure the kidneys and the thyroid are working normally.

Lithium is eliminated from the body through the kidney, so the dose may need to be lowered in older people with reduced kidney function. Also, loss of water from the body, such as through sweating or diarrhea, can cause the lithium level to rise, requiring a temporary lowering of the daily dose. Although kidney functions are checked periodically during lithium treatment, actual damage of the kidney is uncommon in people whose blood levels of lithium have stayed within the therapeutic range.

Some possible side effects linked anticonvulsants (such as valproic acid) include:

- Drowsiness

- Dizziness

- Headache

- Diarrhea

- Constipation

- Changes in appetite

- Weight changes

- Back pain

- Agitation

- Mood swings

- Abnormal thinking

- Uncontrollable shaking of a part of the body

- Loss of coordination

- Uncontrollable movements of the eyes

- Blurred or double vision

- Ringing in the ears

- Hair loss

These medications may also:

- Cause damage to the liver or pancreas, so people taking it should see their doctors regularly

- Increase testosterone (a male hormone) levels in teenage girls and lead to a condition called polycystic ovarian syndrome (a disease that can affect fertility and make the menstrual cycle become irregular)

Medications for common adult health problems, such as diabetes, high blood pressure, anxiety, and depression may interact badly with anticonvulsants. In this case, a doctor can offer other medication options.

Chapter 53

Antidepressant Medications For Children And Adolescents

Depression

Depression is a serious disorder that can cause significant problems in mood, thinking, and behavior at home, in school, and with peers. It is estimated that major depressive disorder (MDD) affects about 5 percent of adolescents.

Treatment For Depression

Research has shown that, as in adults, depression in children and adolescents is treatable. Certain antidepressant medications, called selective serotonin reuptake inhibitors (SSRIs), can be beneficial to children and adolescents with MDD. Certain types of psychological therapies also have been shown to be effective. However, our knowledge of antidepressant treatments in youth, though growing substantially, is limited compared to what we know about treating depression in adults.

There has been some concern that the use of antidepressant medications themselves may induce suicidal behavior in youths. Following a thorough and comprehensive review of all the available published and unpublished controlled clinical trials of antidepressants in children and adolescents, the U.S. Food and Drug Administration (FDA) issued a public warning in October 2004 about an increased risk of suicidal thoughts or behavior (suicidality) in children and adolescents treated with SSRI antidepressant medications. In 2006, an advisory committee to the FDA recommended that the agency extend the warning to include young adults up to age 25.

About This Chapter: This chapter includes text excerpted from "Antidepressant Medications For Children And Adolescents: Information For Parents And Caregivers," National Institute of Mental Health (NIMH), January 13, 2010. Reviewed July 2017.

Results of a comprehensive review of pediatric trials conducted between 1988 and 2006 suggested that the benefits of antidepressant medications likely outweigh their risks to children and adolescents with major depression and anxiety disorders. The study, partially funded by National Institute of Mental Health (NIMH), was published in the April 18, 2007, issue of the Journal of the American Medical Association (JAMA).

What Did The U.S. Food and Drug Administration (FDA) Review Find?

In the FDA review, no completed suicides occurred among nearly 2,200 children treated with SSRI medications. However, about 4 percent of those taking SSRI medications experienced suicidal thinking or behavior, including actual suicide attempts—twice the rate of those taking placebo, or sugar pills.

In response, the FDA adopted a "black box" label warning indicating that antidepressants may increase the risk of suicidal thinking and behavior in some children and adolescents with MDD. A black-box warning is the most serious type of warning in prescription drug labeling.

The warning also notes that children and adolescents taking SSRI medications should be closely monitored for any worsening in depression, emergence of suicidal thinking or behavior, or unusual changes in behavior, such as sleeplessness, agitation, or withdrawal from normal social situations. Close monitoring is especially important during the first four weeks of treatment. SSRI medications usually have few side effects in children and adolescents, but for unknown reasons, they may trigger agitation and abnormal behavior in certain individuals.

What Do We Know About Antidepressant Medications?

The SSRIs include:

- fluoxetine (Prozac)
- citalopram (Celexa)
- sertraline (Zoloft)
- escitalopram (Lexapro)
- paroxetine (Paxil)
- fluvoxamine (Luvox)

Another antidepressant medication, venlafaxine (Effexor), is not an SSRI but is closely related. SSRI medications are considered an improvement over older antidepressant medications because they have fewer side effects and are less likely to be harmful if taken in an overdose, which is an issue for patients with depression already at risk for suicide. They have been shown to be safe and effective for adults.

However, use of SSRI medications among children and adolescents ages 10 to 19 has risen dramatically in the past several years. Fluoxetine (Prozac) is the only medication approved by the FDA for use in treating depression in children ages 8 and older. The other SSRI medications and the SSRI-related antidepressant venlafaxine have not been approved for treatment of depression in children or adolescents, but doctors still sometimes prescribe them to children on an "off-label" basis. In June 2003, however, the FDA recommended that paroxetine not be used in children and adolescents for treating MDD.

Fluoxetine can be helpful in treating childhood depression, and can lead to significant improvement of depression overall. However, it may increase the risk for suicidal behaviors in a small subset of adolescents. As with all medical decisions, doctors and families should weigh the risks and benefits of treatment for each individual patient.

What is the most important information I should know about antidepressant medicines, depression and other serious mental illnesses, and suicidal thoughts or actions?

- Antidepressant medicines may increase suicidal thoughts or actions in some children, teenagers, and young adults when the medicine is first started.

- Depression and other serious mental illnesses are the most important causes of suicidal thoughts and actions. Some people may have a particularly high risk of having suicidal thoughts or actions. These include people who have (or have a family history of) bipolar illness (also called manic-depressive illness) or suicidal thoughts or actions.

What else do I need to know about antidepressant medicines?

- **Never stop an antidepressant medicine without first talking to a healthcare provider.** Stopping an antidepressant medicine suddenly can cause other symptoms.

- **Antidepressants are medicines used to treat depression and other illnesses.** It is important to discuss all the risks of treating depression and also the risks of not treating it. Patients and their families or other caregivers should discuss all treatment choices with the healthcare provider, not just the use of antidepressants.

- **Antidepressant medicines have other side effects.** Talk to the healthcare provider about the side effects of the medicine prescribed for you or your family member.

- **Antidepressant medicines can interact with other medicines.** Know all of the medicines that you or your family member takes. Keep a list of all medicines to show the healthcare provider. Do not start new medicines without first checking with your healthcare provider.

- **Not all antidepressant medicines prescribed for children are FDA approved for use in children**. Talk to your child's healthcare provider for more information.

(Source: "Medication Guide Antidepressant Medicines, Depression And Other Serious Mental Illnesses, Suicidal Thoughts Or Actions," U.S. Food and Drug Administration (FDA).)

What Should You Do For A Child With Depression?

A child or adolescent with MDD should be carefully and thoroughly evaluated by a doctor to determine if medication is appropriate. Psychotherapy often is tried as an initial treatment for mild depression. Psychotherapy may help to determine the severity and persistence of the depression and whether antidepressant medications may be warranted. Types of psychotherapies include "cognitive behavioral therapy," which helps people learn new ways of thinking and behaving, and "interpersonal therapy," which helps people understand and work through troubled personal relationships.

Those who are prescribed an SSRI medication should receive ongoing medical monitoring. Children already taking an SSRI medication should remain on the medication if it has been helpful, but should be carefully monitored by a doctor for side effects. Parents should promptly seek medical advice and evaluation if their child or adolescent experiences suicidal thinking or behavior, nervousness, agitation, irritability, mood instability, or sleeplessness that either emerges or worsens during treatment with SSRI medications.

Once started, treatment with these medications should not be abruptly stopped. Although they are not habit-forming or addictive, abruptly ending an antidepressant can cause withdrawal symptoms or lead to a relapse. Families should not discontinue treatment without consulting their doctor.

All treatments can be associated with side effects. Families and doctors should carefully weigh the risks and benefits, and maintain appropriate follow-up and monitoring to help control for the risks.

Chapter 54

Brain Stimulation Therapies

Brain stimulation therapies can play a role in treating certain mental disorders. Brain stimulation therapies involve activating or inhibiting the brain directly with electricity. The electricity can be given directly by electrodes implanted in the brain, or noninvasively through electrodes placed on the scalp. The electricity can also be induced by using magnetic fields applied to the head. While these types of therapies are less frequently used than medication and psychotherapies, they hold promise for treating certain mental disorders that do not respond to other treatments.

Electroconvulsive therapy (ECT) is the best studied brain stimulation therapy and has the longest history of use. Other stimulation therapies discussed here are newer, and in some cases still experimental methods. These include the following:

- Vagus nerve stimulation (VNS)

- Repetitive transcranial magnetic stimulation (rTMS)

- Magnetic seizure therapy (MST)

- Deep brain stimulation (DBS)

A treatment plan may also include medication and psychotherapy. Choosing the right treatment plan should be based on a person's individual needs and medical situation, and under a doctor's care.

About This Chapter: This chapter includes text excerpted from "Brain Stimulation Therapies," National Institute of Mental Health (NIMH), June 2016.

Electroconvulsive Therapy (ECT)

Electroconvulsive therapy (ECT) uses an electric current to treat serious mental disorders. This type of therapy is usually considered only if a patient's illness has not improved after other treatments (such as antidepressant medication or psychotherapy) are tried, or in cases where rapid response is needed (as in the case of suicide risk and catatonia, for example).

Why It's Done

ECT is most often used to treat severe, treatment-resistant depression, but it may also be medically indicated in other mental disorders, such as bipolar disorder or schizophrenia. It also may be used in life-threatening circumstances, such as when a patient is unable to move or respond to the outside world (e.g., catatonia), is suicidal, or is malnourished as a result of severe depression. ECT can be effective in reducing the chances of relapse when patients undergo follow-up treatments. Two major advantages of ECT over medication are that ECT begins to work quicker, often starting within the first week, and older individuals respond especially quickly.

How It Works

Before ECT is administered, a person is sedated with general anesthesia and given a medication called a muscle relaxant to prevent movement during the procedure. An anesthesiologist monitors breathing, heart rate and blood pressure during the entire procedure, which is conducted by a trained medical team, including physicians and nurses. During the procedure:

- Electrodes are placed at precise locations on the head.

- Through the electrodes, an electric current passes through the brain, causing a seizure that lasts generally less than one minute. Because the patient is under anesthesia and has taken a muscle relaxant, it is not painful and the patient cannot feel the electrical impulses.

- Five to ten minutes after the procedure ends, the patient awakens. He or she may feel groggy at first as the anesthesia wears off. But after about an hour, the patient usually is alert and can resume normal activities.

A typical course of ECT is administered about three times a week until the patient's depression improves (usually within 6 to 12 treatments). After that, maintenance ECT treatment is sometimes needed to reduce the chances that symptoms will return. ECT maintenance treatment varies depending on the needs of the individual, and may range from one session per week to one session every few months. Frequently, a person who undergoes ECT also takes antidepressant medication or a mood stabilizing medication.

Side Effects

The most common side effects associated with ECT include:

- headache

- upset stomach

- muscle aches

- memory loss

Some people may experience memory problems, especially of memories around the time of the treatment. Sometimes the memory problems are more severe, but usually they improve over the days and weeks following the end of an ECT course.

Research has found that memory problems seem to be more associated with the traditional type of ECT called bilateral ECT, in which the electrodes are placed on both sides of the head.

In unilateral ECT, the electrodes are placed on just one side of the head—typically the right side because it is opposite the brain's learning and memory areas. Unilateral ECT has been found to be less likely to cause memory problems and therefore is preferred by many doctors, patients and families.

There are a lot of outdated beliefs about ECT, but based on the latest research,

- ECT can provide relief for people with severe depression who have not been able to feel better with other treatments.

- ECT can be an effective treatment for depression. In some severe cases where a rapid response is necessary, or medications cannot be used safely, ECT can even be a first-line intervention.

- ECT may cause some side effects, including confusion, disorientation, and memory loss. Usually these side effects are short term, but sometimes they can linger.

- Advances in ECT devices and methods have made modern ECT safe and effective for the vast majority of patients.

- Talk to your doctor and make sure you understand the potential benefits and risks of the treatment before giving your informed consent to undergoing ECT.

(Source: "Depression: Electroconvulsive Therapy And Other Brain Stimulation Therapies," NIHSeniorHealth, National Institute on Aging (NIA).)

Vagus Nerve Stimulation (VNS)

Vagus nerve stimulation (VNS) works through a device implanted under the skin that sends electrical pulses through the left vagus nerve, half of a prominent pair of nerves that run from the brainstem through the neck and down to each side of the chest and abdomen. The vagus nerves carry messages from the brain to the body's major organs (e.g., heart, lungs and intestines) and to areas of the brain that control mood, sleep, and other functions.

Why It's Done

VNS was originally developed as a treatment for epilepsy. However, scientists noticed that it also had favorable effects on mood, especially depressive symptoms. Using brain scans, scientists found that the device affected areas of the brain that are involved in mood regulation. The pulses appeared to alter the levels of certain neurotransmitters (brain chemicals) associated with mood, including serotonin, norepinephrine, gamma-aminobutyric acid (GABA), and glutamate.

In 2005, the U.S. Food and Drug Administration (FDA) approved VNS for use in treating treatment-resistant depression in certain circumstances:

- If the patient is 18 years of age or over; and

- If the illness has lasted two years or more; and

- if it is severe or recurrent; and

- if the depression has not eased after trying at least four other treatments

According to the FDA, it is not intended to be a first-line treatment, even for patients with severe depression.

How It Works

A device called a pulse generator, about the size of a stopwatch, is surgically implanted in the upper left side of the chest. Connected to the pulse generator is an electrical lead wire, which is connected from the generator to the left vagus nerve.

Typically, 30-second electrical pulses are sent about every five minutes from the generator to the vagus nerve. The duration and frequency of the pulses may vary depending on how the generator is programmed. The vagus nerve, in turn, delivers those signals to the brain. The pulse generator, which operates continuously, is powered by a battery that lasts around 10 years, after which it must be replaced. Normally, people do not feel pain or any other sensations as the device operates.

The device also can be temporarily deactivated by placing a magnet over the chest where the pulse generator is implanted. A person may want to deactivate it if side effects become intolerable, or before engaging in strenuous activity or exercise because it may interfere with breathing. The device reactivates when the magnet is removed.

> VNS should only be prescribed and monitored by doctors who have specific training and expertise in the management of treatment-resistant depression and the use of this device.

VNS treatment is intended to reduce symptoms of depression. It may be several months before the patient notices any benefits and not all patients will respond to VNS. It is important to remember that VNS is intended to be given along with other traditional therapies, such as medications, and patients should not expect to discontinue these other treatments, even with the device in place.

Side Effects

VNS is not without risk. There may be complications such as infection from the implant surgery, or the device may come loose, move around or malfunction, which may require additional surgery to correct. Some patients have no improvement in symptoms and some actually get worse.

Other potential side effects include:

- Voice changes or hoarseness
- Cough or sore throat
- Neck pain
- Discomfort or tingling in the area where the device is implanted
- Breathing problems, especially during exercise
- Difficulty swallowing

Long-term side effects are unknown.

Repetitive Transcranial Magnetic Stimulation (rTMS)

Repetitive transcranial magnetic stimulation (rTMS) uses a magnet to activate the brain. First developed in 1985, rTMS has been studied as a treatment for depression, psychosis, anxiety, and other disorders.

Unlike ECT, in which electrical stimulation is more generalized, rTMS can be targeted to a specific site in the brain. Scientists believe that focusing on a specific site in the brain reduces the chance for the types of side effects associated with ECT. But opinions vary as to what site is best.

Why It's Done

In 2008, rTMS was approved for use by the FDA as a treatment for major depression for patients who do not respond to at least one antidepressant medication in the current episode. It is also used in other countries as a treatment for depression in patients who have not responded to medications and who might otherwise be considered for ECT.

The evidence supporting rTMS for depression was mixed until the first large clinical trial, funded by National Institute of Mental Health (NIMH), was published in 2010. The trial found that 14 percent achieved remission with rTMS compared to 5 percent with an inactive (sham) treatment. After the trial ended, patients could enter a second phase in which everyone, including those who previously received the sham treatment, was given rTMS. Remission rates during the second phase climbed to nearly 30 percent. A sham treatment is like a placebo, but instead of being an inactive pill, it's an inactive procedure that mimics real rTMS.

How It Works

A typical rTMS session lasts 30 to 60 minutes and does not require anesthesia.

During the procedure:

- An electromagnetic coil is held against the forehead near an area of the brain that is thought to be involved in mood regulation.

- Then, short electromagnetic pulses are administered through the coil. The magnetic pulses easily pass through the skull, and causes small electrical currents that stimulate nerve cells in the targeted brain region.

Because this type of pulse generally does not reach further than two inches into the brain, scientists can select which parts of the brain will be affected and which will not be. The magnetic field is about the same strength as that of a magnetic resonance imaging (MRI) scan. Generally, the person feels a slight knocking or tapping on the head as the pulses are administered.

Not all scientists agree on the best way to position the magnet on the patient's head or give the electromagnetic pulses. They also do not yet know if rTMS works best when given as a single treatment or combined with medication and/or psychotherapy.

Side Effects

Sometimes a person may have discomfort at the site on the head where the magnet is placed. The muscles of the scalp, jaw or face may contract or tingle during the procedure. Mild headaches or brief lightheadedness may result. It is also possible that the procedure could cause a seizure, although documented incidences of this are uncommon. Two large-scale studies on the safety of rTMS found that most side effects, such as headaches or scalp discomfort, were mild or moderate, and no seizures occurred. Because the treatment is relatively new, however, long-term side effects are unknown.

Magnetic Seizure Therapy (MST)

How It Works

Magnetic seizure therapy (MST) borrows certain aspects from both ECT and rTMS. Like rTMS, MST uses magnetic pulses instead of electricity to stimulate a precise target in the brain. However, unlike rTMS, MST aims to induce a seizure like ECT. So the pulses are given at a higher frequency than that used in rTMS. Therefore, like ECT, the patient must be anesthetized and given a muscle relaxant to prevent movement. The goal of MST is to retain the effectiveness of ECT while reducing its cognitive side effects.

MST is in the early stages of testing for mental disorders, but initial results are promising. A recent review article that examined the evidence from eight clinical studies found that MST triggered remission from major depression or bipolar disorder in 30–40 percent of individuals.

Side Effects

Like ECT, MST carries the risk of side effects that can be caused by anesthesia exposure and the induction of a seizure. Studies in both animals and humans have found that MST produces

- fewer memory side effects

- shorter seizures

- allows for a shorter recovery time than ECT

Deep Brain Stimulation (DBS)

Deep brain stimulation (DBS) was first developed as a treatment for Parkinson disease to reduce tremor, stiffness, walking problems, and uncontrollable movements. In DBS, a pair of electrodes is implanted in the brain and controlled by a generator that is implanted in the chest. Stimulation is continuous and its frequency and level are customized to the individual.

DBS has been studied as a treatment for depression or obsessive-compulsive disorder (OCD). Currently, there is a Humanitarian Device Exemption for the use of DBS to treat OCD, but its use in depression remains only on an experimental basis. A review of all 22 published studies testing DBS for depression found that only three of them were of high quality because they not only had a treatment group but also a control group which did not receive DBS. The review found that across the studies, 40–50 percent of people showed receiving DBS greater than 50 percent improvement.

How It Works

DBS requires brain surgery. The head is shaved and then attached with screws to a sturdy frame that prevents the head from moving during the surgery. Scans of the head and brain using MRI are taken. The surgeon uses these images as guides during the surgery. Patients are awake during the procedure to provide the surgeon with feedback, but they feel no pain because the head is numbed with a local anesthetic and the brain itself does not register pain.

Once ready for surgery, two holes are drilled into the head. From there, the surgeon threads a slender tube down into the brain to place electrodes on each side of a specific area of the brain. In the case of depression, the first area of the brain targeted by DBS is called Area 25, or the subgenual cingulate cortex. This area has been found to be overactive in depression and other mood disorders. But later research targeted several other areas of the brain affected by depression. So DBS is now targeting several areas of the brain for treating depression. In the case of OCD, the electrodes are placed in an area of the brain (the ventral capsule/ventral striatum) believed to be associated with the disorder.

After the electrodes are implanted and the patient provides feedback about their placement, the patient is put under general anesthesia. The electrodes are then attached to wires that are run inside the body from the head down to the chest, where a pair of battery-operated generators are implanted. From here, electrical pulses are continuously delivered over the wires to the electrodes in the brain. Although it is unclear exactly how the device works to reduce depression or OCD, scientists believe that the pulses help to "reset" the area of the brain that is malfunctioning so that it works normally again.

Side Effects

DBS carries risks associated with any type of brain surgery. For example, the procedure may lead to:

- Bleeding in the brain or stroke

- Infection

- Disorientation or confusion

- Unwanted mood changes

- Movement disorders

- Lightheadedness

- Trouble sleeping

Because the procedure is still being studied, other side effects not yet identified may be possible. Long-term benefits and side effects are unknown.

Chapter 55

Complementary And Alternative Approaches To Mental Healthcare

Complementary And Alternative Medicine (CAM)

Complementary and alternative medicine (CAM) is a group of diverse medical and health-care systems, practices, and products that are not generally considered part of conventional medicine. Complementary medicine is used together with conventional medicine, and alternative medicine is used in place of conventional medicine. Integrative medicine combines conventional and CAM treatments for which there is evidence of safety and effectiveness. While scientific evidence exists regarding some CAM therapies, for most there are key questions that are yet to be answered through well-designed scientific studies—questions such as whether these therapies are safe and whether they work for the purposes for which they are used.

Complementary Versus Alternative

Many Americans—more than 30 percent of adults and about 12 percent of children—use healthcare approaches developed outside of mainstream Western, or conventional, medicine. When describing these approaches, people often use "alternative" and "complementary" interchangeably, but the two terms refer to different concepts:

About This Chapter: Text under the heading "Complementary And Alternative Medicine (CAM)" is excerpted from "The Use Of Complementary And Alternative Medicine In The United States," National Center for Complementary and Integrative Health (NCCIH), March 22, 2016; Text under the heading "Relaxation Techniques" is excerpted from "Relaxation Techniques For Health," National Center for Complementary and Integrative Health (NCCIH), April 20, 2017; Text under the heading "Meditation" is excerpted from "Meditation: In Depth," National Center for Complementary and Integrative Health (NCCIH), March 17, 2017; Text under the heading "Natural Products For Depression" is excerpted from "Depression And Complementary Health Approaches: What The Science Says," National Center for Complementary and Integrative Health (NCCIH), April 22, 2016.

> - If a non-mainstream practice is used together with conventional medicine, it's considered "complementary."
> - If a non-mainstream practice is used in place of conventional medicine, it's considered "alternative."
>
> True alternative medicine is uncommon. Most people who use non-mainstream approaches use them along with conventional treatments.
>
> *(Source: "Complementary, Alternative, Or Integrative Health: What's In A Name?" National Center for Complementary and Alternative Medicine (NCCAM).)*

Relaxation Techniques

What Are Relaxation Techniques?

Relaxation techniques include a number of practices such as progressive relaxation, guided imagery, biofeedback, self-hypnosis, and deep breathing exercises. The goal is similar in all:

- to produce the body's natural relaxation response,
- characterized by slower breathing,
- lower blood pressure, and
- a feeling of increased well-being.

Meditation and practices that include meditation with movement, such as yoga and tai chi, can also promote relaxation. Stress management programs commonly include relaxation techniques. Relaxation techniques have also been studied to see whether they might be of value in managing various health problems.

What The Science Says About The Effectiveness Of Relaxation Techniques

Researchers have evaluated relaxation techniques to see whether they could play a role in managing a variety of health conditions, including the following:

Anxiety

Studies have shown relaxation techniques may reduce anxiety in people with ongoing health problems such as heart disease or inflammatory bowel disease, and in those who are having medical procedures such as breast biopsies or dental treatment. Relaxation techniques have also been shown to be useful for older adults with anxiety.

On the other hand, relaxation techniques may not be the best way to help people with generalized anxiety disorder. Generalized anxiety disorder is a mental health condition, lasting for months or longer, in which a person is often worried or anxious about many things and finds it hard to control the anxiety. Studies indicate that long-term results are better in people with generalized anxiety disorder who receive a type of psychotherapy called cognitive-behavioral therapy than in those who are taught relaxation techniques.

Depression

An evaluation of 15 studies concluded that relaxation techniques are better than no treatment in reducing symptoms of depression but are not as beneficial as psychological therapies such as cognitive-behavioral therapy.

Insomnia

There's evidence that relaxation techniques can be helpful in managing chronic insomnia. Relaxation techniques can be combined with other strategies for getting a good night's sleep, such as maintaining a consistent sleep schedule; avoiding caffeine, alcohol, heavy meals, and strenuous exercise too close to bedtime; and sleeping in a quiet, cool, dark room.

Nightmares

Some studies have indicated that relaxation exercises may be an effective approach for nightmares of unknown cause and those associated with posttraumatic stress disorder. However, an assessment of many studies concluded that relaxation is less helpful than more extensive forms of treatment (psychotherapy or medication).

What The Science Says About The Safety And Side Effects Of Relaxation Techniques

Relaxation techniques are generally considered safe for healthy people. However, occasionally, people report negative experiences such as increased anxiety, intrusive thoughts, or fear of losing control.

There have been rare reports that certain relaxation techniques might cause or worsen symptoms in people with epilepsy or certain psychiatric conditions, or with a history of abuse or trauma. People with heart disease should talk to their healthcare provider before doing progressive muscle relaxation.

Who Teaches Relaxation Techniques?

A variety of professionals, including physicians, psychologists, social workers, nurses, and complementary health practitioners, may teach relaxation techniques. Also, people sometimes learn the simpler relaxation techniques on their own.

Meditation

What Is Medication?

Meditation is a mind and body practice that has a long history of use for increasing calmness and physical relaxation, improving psychological balance, coping with illness, and enhancing overall health and well-being. Mind and body practices focus on the interactions among the brain, mind, body, and behavior.

There are many types of meditation, but most have four elements in common:

1. a quiet location with as few distractions as possible;

2. a specific, comfortable posture (sitting, lying down, walking, or in other positions);

3. a focus of attention (a specially chosen word or set of words, an object, or the sensations of the breath); and

4. an open attitude (letting distractions come and go naturally without judging them).

What The Science Says About The Effectiveness Of Meditation

Many studies have investigated meditation for different conditions, and there's evidence that it may reduce blood pressure as well as symptoms of irritable bowel syndrome and flare-ups in people who have had ulcerative colitis. It may ease symptoms of anxiety and depression, and may help people with insomnia.

Anxiety, Depression, And Insomnia

A 2014 literature review of 47 trials in 3,515 participants suggests that mindfulness meditation programs show moderate evidence of improving anxiety and depression. But the researchers found no evidence that meditation changed health-related behaviors affected by stress, such as substance abuse and sleep.

In a small, NCCIH-funded study, 54 adults with chronic insomnia learned mindfulness-based stress reduction (MBSR), a form of MBSR specially adapted to deal with insomnia (mindfulness-based therapy for insomnia, or MBTI), or a self-monitoring program. Both meditation-based programs aided sleep, with MBTI providing a significantly greater reduction in insomnia severity compared with MBSR.

Other Conditions

Results from a NCCIH-funded study of 279 adults who participated in an 8-week Mindfulness-Based Stress Reduction (MBSR) program found that changes in spirituality were associated with better mental health and quality of life.

Guidelines from the American College of Chest Physicians published in 2013 suggest that MBSR and meditation may help to reduce stress, anxiety, pain, and depression while enhancing mood and self-esteem in people with lung cancer.

Clinical practice guidelines issued in 2014 by the Society for Integrative Oncology (SIC) recommend meditation as supportive care to reduce stress, anxiety, depression, and fatigue in patients treated for breast cancer. The SIC also recommends its use to improve quality of life in these people.

Meditation-based programs may be helpful in reducing common menopausal symptoms, including the frequency and intensity of hot flashes, sleep and mood disturbances, stress, and muscle and joint pain. However, differences in study designs mean that no firm conclusions can be drawn.

Because only a few studies have been conducted on the effects of meditation for attention deficit hyperactivity disorder (ADHD), there isn't sufficient evidence to support its use for this condition.

A 2014 research review suggested that mind and body practices, including meditation, reduce chemical identifiers of inflammation and show promise in helping to regulate the immune system. Results from a 2013 NCCIH-supported study involving 49 adults suggest that 8 weeks of mindfulness training may reduce stress-induced inflammation better than a health program that includes physical activity, education about diet, and music therapy.

Natural Products For Depression

Omega-3 Fatty Acids

Some evidence suggests that omega-3 fatty acid supplementation may provide a small effect in adjunctive therapy in patients with a diagnosis of major depressive disorder (MDD) and on depressive patients without a diagnosis of MDD. Most trials have been adjunctive studies. Although the data are promising, controlled trials of omega-3 fatty acids as a monotherapy are inconclusive compared to standard antidepressant medicines, and it remains unclear that a mechanism is present to suggest that a pharmacological or biological antidepressant effect exists.

St. John's Wort

There is some evidence that suggests St. John's wort *(Hypericum perforatum)* may have an effect on mild to moderate major depressive disorder (MDD) for a limited number of patients, similar to standard antidepressants, but the evidence is far from definitive. Although some studies have demonstrated a slight efficacy over placebo, others contradict these findings.

The significant herb-drug interactions of St. John's wort *(Hypericum perforatum)* are important safety considerations and may outweigh any benefit of its use.

Part Seven
Mental Wellness Topics For Teens

Chapter 56

Building Healthy Self-Esteem

What Is Self-Esteem?

Self-esteem has to do with the value and respect you have for yourself. Simply put, it's your opinion of yourself.

If you have healthy self-esteem, you feel good about yourself and are proud of what you can do. Having healthy self-esteem can help you feel positive overall. And it can make you brave enough to tackle some serious challenges, like trying out for a school play or standing up to a bully.

If you have low self-esteem, you may not think very highly of yourself. Of course, it's normal to feel down about yourself sometimes. But if you feel bad about yourself more often than good, you may have low self-esteem. You can read about rating your self-esteem.

Low self-esteem may stop you from doing things you want to do or from speaking up for yourself. Low self-esteem may even lead you to try to feel better in unhealthy ways, like using drugs or alcohol. Also, some people may start to feel so sad or hopeless about themselves that they develop mental health problems like depression and eating disorders.

A lot of things can affect self-esteem. These include how others treat you, your background and culture, and experiences at school. For example, being put down by your boyfriend,

About This Chapter: Text beginning with the heading "What Is Self-Esteem?" is excerpted from "Self-Esteem And Self-Confidence," girlshealth.gov, Office on Women's Health (OWH), February 11, 2015; Text under the heading "Self-Help Guide To Build Self-Esteem" is excerpted from "Building Self-Esteem: A Self-Help Guide," Substance Abuse and Mental Health Services Administration (SAMHSA), January 2002. Reviewed July 2017; Text under the heading "Ways To Boost Self-Esteem" is excerpted from "Ways To Build Self-Esteem," girlshealth.gov, Office on Women's Health (OWH), December 22, 2015.

classmates, or family or being bullied can affect how you see yourself. But one of the biggest influences on your self-esteem is—you!

Rate Your Self-Esteem

If you have healthy self-esteem and self-confidence, you probably will agree with some or most of the following statements:

- I feel good about who I am.

- I am proud of what I can do, but don't need to show off.

- I know there are some things that I'm good at and some things I need to improve.

- I feel it is okay if I win or if I lose.

- I usually think, "I can do this," before I do something.

- I am eager to learn new things.

- I can handle criticism.

- I like to try to do things without help, but I don't mind asking for help if I need it.

- I like myself.

If some of the items on this checklist are true for you, congrats! You're on the right track. And if your self-esteem ever slips, you can try these steps.

If you have low self-esteem and self-confidence, you probably will agree with some or most of the following statements:

- I can't do anything well.

- I have no friends.

- I do not like to try new things.

- I get really upset about making mistakes.

- I'm not as nice, pretty, or smart as the other girls in my class.

- I don't like it when people say nice things about me.

- I get very upset when people criticize me.

- I feel better if I put other people down.

- I don't know what I'm good at.

- I usually think, "I can't do this," before I do something.
- I don't like myself.

If many of the items on this list apply to you, try some ways to raise your self-esteem. It's no fun to be hard on yourself, and you can work to stop. Remember, everyone brings something unique to the world.

Self-Help Guide To Build Self-Esteem

Most people feel bad about themselves from time to time. Feelings of low self-esteem may be triggered by being treated poorly by someone else recently or in the past, or by a person's own judgments of him or herself. This is normal. However, low self-esteem is a constant companion for too many people, especially those who experience depression, anxiety, phobias, psychosis, delusional thinking, or who have an illness or a disability. If you are one of these people, you may go through life feeling bad about yourself needlessly. Low self-esteem keeps you from enjoying life, doing the things you want to do, and working toward personal goals.

You have a right to feel good about yourself. However, it can be very difficult to feel good about yourself when you are under the stress of having symptoms that are hard to manage, when you are dealing with a disability, when you are having a difficult time, or when others are treating you badly. At these times, it is easy to be drawn into a downward spiral of lower and lower self- esteem. For instance, you may begin feeling bad about yourself when someone insults you, you are under a lot of pressure at work, or you are having a difficult time getting along with someone in your family. Then you begin to give yourself negative self-talk, like "I'm no good." That may make you feel so bad about yourself that you do something to hurt yourself or someone else, such as getting drunk or yelling at your children.

Things You Can Do Right Away—Every Day—To Build Your Self-Esteem

- Pay attention to your own needs and wants.
- Take very good care of yourself.
- Take time to do things you enjoy.
- Get something done that you have been putting off.
- Do things that make use of your own special talents and abilities.
- Dress in clothes that make you feel good about yourself.

- Give yourself rewards.

- Spend time with people who make you feel good about yourself—people who treat you well. Avoid people who treat you badly

- Make your living space a place that honors the person you are.

- Display items that you find attractive or that remind you of your achievements or of special times or people in your life

- Make your meals a special time. Turn off the television, radio, and stereo. Set the table, even if you are eating alone. Light a candle or put some flowers or an attractive object in the center of the table. Arrange your food in an attractive way on your plate. If you eat with others, encourage discussion of pleasant topics. Avoid discussing difficult issues at meals.

- Take advantage of opportunities to learn something new or improve your skills. Take a class or go to a seminar. Many adult education programs are free or very inexpensive. For those that are more costly, ask about a possible scholarship or fee reduction.

- Begin doing those things that you know will make you feel better about yourself—like going on a diet, beginning an exercise program or keeping your living space clean.

- Do something nice for another person. Smile at someone who looks sad. Say a few kind words to the check-out cashier. Help your spouse with an unpleasant chore. Take a meal to a friend who is sick. Send a card to an acquaintance. Volunteer for a worthy organization.

- Make it a point to treat yourself well every day. Before you go to bed each night, write about how you treated yourself well during the day.

Ways To Boost Self-Esteem

Having healthy or high self-esteem means that you feel good about yourself and are proud of what you can do. Having high self-esteem can help you to think positively, deal better with stress, and boost your drive to work hard. Having high self-esteem can also make it easier to try new things. Before you try something new, you think, "I can do this," and not, "This is too hard. I'll never be able to do this."

If you have an illness or disability, how does it affect your self-esteem? Do you find your self-esteem is affected by how you think others see you? Do people put you down or bully you? This can put your self-esteem at risk. If you need a self-esteem boost, take these steps:

- Ask yourself what you are really good at and enjoy doing. Everyone is good at something. When you're feeling bad about yourself, just think, "I'm good at art" (or computers or playing an instrument or whatever you're good at). You might make a list of your great traits and talents, too. And remember that it's okay not to be great at everything.

- Push yourself to try new things. If you try something new and fail, that's okay. Everyone fails sometime. Try to figure out what went wrong, so you can try again in a new way. Keep trying, and don't give up. In time, you'll figure out how to succeed.

- Always give your best effort, and take pride in your effort. When you accomplish a goal, celebrate over a family meal or treat yourself to a fun outing.

- If you need help, ask for it. Talking to a parent, teacher, or friend can help you come up with different ways to solve a problem. This is called brainstorming. Make a list of your possible solutions. Put the ones that you think will work the best at the top. Then rehearse them ahead of time so that you'll know exactly what you're going to do or say when the problem comes up. If your first plan doesn't work, then go on to Plan B. If Plan B doesn't work, go on to Plan C, and so on.

- Join a support group. Finding out how other kids deal with illnesses or disabilities can help you cope. Ask your doctor, teachers, or parents for help finding a support group in your community or online. Check out these options for chatting with other kids online. Make sure to get your parent's permission first.

- Volunteer to do something at school or in your community. For instance, you could tutor a younger child or take care of the plants in the community center lobby. You might also volunteer to do some chores at home.

- Look for ways to take more control over your life. For instance, every student who has needs related to an illness or disability in school must have an Individualized Education Plan, or IEP. Your IEP describes your goals during the school year and any support that you'll need to help achieve those goals. Get involved with the development of your IEP. Attend any IEP meetings. Tell your parents, teachers, and others involved in your IEP what you think your goals at school should be and what would help you achieve them. It's your education, and you get a say in what happens! Learn more about the Individualized Education Plan External link.

- Speak up for yourself. This can be difficult if you're shy. But it can get easier with practice. Learn to communicate your needs and don't hesitate to ask for something.

- Work on trying to feel good about how you look. Everyone has some things they like and don't like about their bodies. It pays to focus on the positives since your body image, or how you feel about your looks, can affect your self-esteem. And remember that real beauty comes from the inside! If you like makeup and clothes, ask for help dealing with any obstacles your illness or disability might present.

- If you still find that you are not feeling good about yourself, talk to your parents, a school counselor, or your doctor because you may be at risk for depression. You can also ask the school nurse if your school offers counseling for help through tough times.

Chapter 57

Improving Mental Health

Your mental health is very important. You will not have a healthy body if you don't also take care of your mind. It's important for you to take care of yourself so that you can do the important things in life—whether it's working, learning, taking care of your family, volunteering, enjoying the outdoors, or whatever is important to you.

Good mental health helps you enjoy life and cope with problems. It offers a feeling of well-being and inner strength. Just as you take care of your body by eating right and exercising, you can do things to protect your mental health. In fact, eating right and exercising can help maintain good mental health. You don't automatically have good mental health just because you don't have mental health illness. You have to work to keep your mind healthy.

Nutrition And Mental Health

The food you eat can have a direct effect on your energy level, physical health, and mood. A "healthy diet" is one that has enough of each essential nutrient, contains many foods from all of the basic food groups, provides the right amount of calories to maintain a healthy weight, and does not have too much fat, sugar, salt, or alcohol.

By choosing foods that can give you steady energy, you can help your body stay healthy. This may also help your mind feel good. The same diet doesn't work for every person. In order to find the best foods that are right for you, talk to your healthcare professional.

About This Chapter: This chapter includes text excerpted from "Good Mental Health," Office on Women's Health (OWH), U.S. Department of Health and Human Services (HHS), March 29, 2010. Reviewed July 2017.

Visit www.choosemyplate.gov to help find personalized eating plans and other interactive tools to help you make good food choices.

Some vitamins and minerals may help with the symptoms of depression. Experts are looking into how a lack of some nutrients—including folate, vitamin B12, calcium, iron, selenium, zinc, and omega-3—may contribute to depression in new mothers. Ask your doctor or another healthcare professional for more information.

Exercise And Mental Health

Regular physical activity is important to the physical and mental health of almost everyone, including older adults. Being physically active can help you continue to do the things you enjoy and stay independent as you age. Regular physical activity over long periods of time can produce long-term health benefits. That's why health experts say that everyone should be active every day to maintain their health.

If you are diagnosed with depression or anxiety, your doctor may tell you to exercise in addition to taking any medications or receiving counseling. This is because exercise has been shown to help with the symptoms of depression and anxiety. Your body makes certain chemicals, called endorphins, before and after you work out. They relieve stress and improve your mood. Exercise can also slow or stop weight gain, which is a common side effect of some medications used to treat mental health disorders.

Regular physical activity can help keep your thinking, learning, and judgment skills sharp as you age. It can also reduce your risk of depression and may help you sleep better. Research has shown that doing aerobic or a mix of aerobic and muscle-strengthening activities 3 to 5 times a week for 30 to 60 minutes can give you these mental health benefits. Some scientific evidence has also shown that even lower levels of physical activity can be beneficial.

(Source: "Physical Activity And Health," Centers for Disease Control and Prevention (CDC).)

Sleep And Mental Health

Your mind and body will feel better if you sleep well. Your body needs time every day to rest and heal. If you often have trouble sleeping—either falling asleep, or waking during the night and being unable to get back to sleep—one or several of the following ideas might be helpful to you:

- Go to bed at the same time every night and get up at the same time every morning. Avoid "sleeping in" (sleeping much later than your usual time for getting up). It will make you feel worse.

- Establish a bedtime "ritual" by doing the same things every night for an hour or two before bedtime so your body knows when it is time to go to sleep.

- Avoid caffeine.

- Eat on a regular schedule and avoid a heavy meal prior to going to bed. Don't skip any meals.

- Eat plenty of dairy foods and dark green leafy vegetables.

- Exercise daily, but avoid strenuous or invigorating activity before going to bed.

- Play soothing music on a tape or compact disc (CD) that shuts off automatically after you are in bed.

- Try a turkey sandwich and a glass of milk before bedtime to make you feel drowsy.

- Try having a small snack before you go to bed, something like a piece of fruit and a piece of cheese, so you don't wake up hungry in the middle of the night. Have a similar small snack if you awaken in the middle of the night.

- Take a warm bath or shower before going to bed.

- Don't smoke.

- Don't drink alcohol.

You need to see your doctor if:

- You often have difficulty sleeping and the solutions listed above are not working for you.

- You awaken during the night gasping for breath.

- Your partner says that your breathing stops when you are sleeping.

- You snore loudly.

- You wake up feeling like you haven't been asleep.

- You fall asleep often during the day.

Stress And Mental Health

Stress can happen for many reasons. Stress can be brought about by a traumatic accident, death, or emergency situation. Stress can also be a side effect of a serious illness or disease.

There is also stress associated with daily life, the workplace, and family responsibilities. It's hard to stay calm and relaxed in our hectic lives. As women, we have many roles: spouse, mother, caregiver, friend, and/or worker. With all we have going on in our lives, it seems almost impossible to find ways to de-stress. But it's important to find those ways. Your health depends on it.

Common symptoms include:

- Headache

- Sleep disorders

- Difficulty concentrating

- Short-temper

- Upset stomach

- Job dissatisfaction

- Low morale

- Depression

- Anxiety

Remember to always make time for you. It's important to care for yourself. Think of this as an order from your doctor, so you don't feel guilty! No matter how busy you are, you can try to set aside at least 15 minutes each day in your schedule to do something for yourself, like taking a bubble bath, going for a walk, or calling a friend.

Chapter 58

Dealing With Depression: Self-Help And Coping Tips

Depression is a serious medical illness and an important public health issue. Depression is characterized by persistent sadness and sometimes irritability (particularly in children) and is one of the leading causes of disease or injury worldwide for both men and women. Depression can cause suffering for depressed individuals and can also have negative effects on their families and the communities in which they live. Depression is associated with significant healthcare needs, school problems, loss of work, and earlier mortality.

Depression

- Is associated with an increased risk for mortality from suicide as well as other causes, such as heart disease

- Is associated with lower workplace productivity and more absenteeism, which result in lower income and higher unemployment.

- Is associated with higher risk for other conditions and behaviors, including:

  - Other mental disorders (anxiety disorders, substance use disorders, eating disorders)

  - Smoking

Although effective treatments are available, many individuals with depression do not have access to treatment or do not take advantage of services. If not effectively treated, depression is likely to become a chronic disease. Just experiencing one episode of depression places an individual at a 50 percent risk for experiencing another episode, and further increases the chances of having more depression episodes in the future.

(Source: "Depression," Centers for Disease Control and Prevention (CDC).)

About This Chapter: This chapter includes text excerpted from "Health Campaigns—Depression," Federal Occupational Health (FOH), U.S. Department of Health and Human Services (HHS), October 12, 2016.

Dealing With Depression

Depression can strongly affect your life. It can drag you down, keeping you from experiencing your full potential. Most people occasionally feel "blue," while clinically depressed people can appear to be functioning normally while just beneath the surface they struggle with feelings of sadness, discouragement, and worthlessness over a prolonged period.

Moving Forward

One of the biggest problems with depression is that it robs you of the energy and motivation necessary to deal effectively with the disorder and move forward.

The first step is realizing that you are depressed. The next step is to take action—and seek help, if you need it—so that you can successfully overcome depression and move on. The most common symptoms of depression include regularly and consistently feeling:

- Sad—"down" or "blue"
- Numb or detached—feeling "empty"
- Hopeless
- Fatigued
- Worthless—low self esteem
- Helpless
- Overwhelmed
- Pessimistic
- Nervous or anxious
- Irritable
- Restless

You, or someone you know, may have one or more of these symptoms. If depression becomes overwhelming, or if it gets in the way of living your life as fully as you would like, talk to your Employee Assistance Program (EAP), a mental health professional, or a physician to start the first steps of moving ahead—and away from depression.

Tips For Avoiding Depression

If your depression is not too serious, you may try some simple things to help avoid biochemical, emotional, and psychological factors that can contribute to the disorder.

- Get plenty of physical activity, especially aerobic activity—brisk walking, running, biking, etc.
- Get quality sleep
- Add more social activity to your week

- Find activities that get you out and make you feel good about yourself—sports teams, adult education classes, etc.

- Avoid alcohol and other recreational drug use—drugs taken to escape or to elevate your mood rather than those used for medicinal purposes

- Volunteer—this can get you "out of yourself"—not as worried about your own problems—and it can get you into a more social environment

- Reprogram negative thought patterns with positive affirmations. For example, rather than allowing a thought like "I'm never happy" or "I wish I were happier" to dominate, you can replace this thought pattern with "I deserve to be happy" and "Everything's going my way now." The affirmation will likely not seem true at first, but as you become more comfortable with the new thought pattern, you'll begin to feel less anxious about these issues.

When To Seek Professional Help

If you continue to suffer from the effects of emotional distress and feel overwhelmed by it, you should contact a professional. Here are some red flags to look out for:

- Inability to sleep

- Feeling down, hopeless, or helpless most of the time

- Concentration problems that are interfering with your work or home life

- Using tobacco, food, drugs, or alcohol to cope with difficult emotions

- Negative or self-destructive thoughts or fears that you can't control*

- Thoughts of death or suicide*

Having self-destructive behavior or thoughts, especially suicidal ones, is a symptom that needs immediate attention. If you experience such feelings and feel that you need help, call your Employee Assistance Program (EAP) or the National Suicide Prevention Lifeline's toll-free number, which is available 24 hours every day of the year: 1–800–273–8255. This service is available to everyone. You may call for yourself or for someone you care about. All calls are confidential.

Chapter 59

Coping With Stress

Physical or emotional tension are often signs of stress. They can be reactions to a situation that cause you to feel threatened or anxious. Stress can be related to positive events (such as planning your wedding) or negative events (such as dealing with the effects of a natural disaster).

Strong emotions like fear, sadness, or other symptoms of depression are normal, as long as they are temporary and don't interfere with daily activities. If these emotions last too long or cause other problems, it's a different story.

Sometimes stress can be good. It can help you develop skills needed to manage potentially threatening situations. Stress can be harmful, however, when it is prolonged or severe enough to make you feel overwhelmed and out of control.

Symptoms Of Stress

Common reactions to a stressful event include:

- Disbelief and shock
- Tension and irritability
- Fear and anxiety about the future
- Difficulty making decisions
- Feeling numb
- Loss of interest in normal activities
- Loss of appetite
- Nightmares and recurring thoughts about the event

About This Chapter: This chapter includes text excerpted from "BAM! Body And Mind—Feelin' Frazzled," Centers for Disease Control and Prevention (CDC), May 9, 2015.

- Anger
- Increased use of alcohol and drugs
- Sadness and other symptoms of depression
- Feeling powerless
- Crying
- Sleep problems
- Headaches, back pains, and stomach problems
- Trouble concentrating

(Source: "Coping With Stress," Centers for Disease Control and Prevention (CDC).)

Finding yourself in a hectic situation, whether it's forgetting your homework or missing your ride home, can really stress you out. Are you looking for a safety net for those days that seem to get worse by the second? Could you really use some advice on how to de-stress both your body and your mind? Knowing how to deal can be half the battle!

Check out these ten tips to keep you cool, calm, and collected:

1. **Put your body in motion.**

   Moving from the chair to the couch while watching TV is not being physically active! Physical activity is one of the most important ways to keep stress away by clearing your head and lifting your spirits. Physical activity also increases endorphin levels—the natural "feel-good" chemicals in the body which leave you with a naturally happy feeling.

   Whether you like full-fledged games of football, tennis, or roller hockey, or you prefer walks with family and friends, it's important to get up, get out, and get moving! Check out the body and mind (BAM)! activity cards and find one that's right for you!

2. **Fuel up.**

   Start your day off with a full tank—eating breakfast will give you the energy you need to tackle the day. Eating regular meals (this means no skipping dinner) and taking time to enjoy them (nope, eating in the car on the way to practice doesn't count) will make you feel better too.

   Make sure to fuel up with fruits, vegetables, proteins, (peanut butter, a chicken sandwich, or a tuna salad) and grains (wheat bread, pasta, or some crackers)—these will give you the power you need to make it through those hectic days.

Don't be fooled by the jolt of energy you get from sodas and sugary snacks—this only lasts a short time, and once it wears off, you may feel sluggish and more tired than usual. For that extra boost of energy to sail through history notes, math class, and after school activities, grab a banana, some string cheese, or a granola bar for some power-packed energy!

3. **Laughing out loud (LOL)!**

    Some say that laughter is the best medicine—well, in many cases, it is! Did you know that it takes 15 facial muscles to laugh? Lots of laughin' can make you feel good—and, that good feeling can stay with you even after the laughter stops. So, head off stress with regular doses of laughter by watching a funny movie or cartoons, reading a joke book (you may even learn some new jokes), or even make up your own riddles—laughter can make you feel like a new person!

    Everyone has those days when they do something really silly or stupid—instead of getting upset with yourself, laugh out loud! No one's perfect! Life should be about having fun. So, lighten up!

4. **Have fun with friends.**

    Being with people you like is always a good way to ditch your stress. Get a group together to go to the movies, shoot some hoops, or play a board game—or just hang out and talk. Friends can help you work through your problems and let you see the brighter side of things.

5. **Spill to someone you trust.**

    Instead of keeping your feelings bottled up inside, talk to someone you trust or respect about what's bothering you. It could be a friend, a parent, someone in your family, or a teacher. Talking out your problems and seeing them from a different view might help you figure out ways to deal with them. Just remember, you don't have to go it alone!

6. **Take time to chill.**

    Pick a comfy spot to sit and read, daydream, or even take a snooze. Listen to your favorite music. Work on a relaxing project like putting together a puzzle or making jewelry.

    Stress can sometimes make you feel like a tight rubber band—stretched to the limit! If this happens, take a few deep breaths to help yourself unwind. If you're in the middle of an impossible homework problem, take a break! Finding time to relax after (and sometimes during) a hectic day or week can make all the difference.

7. **Catch some *zzzzz*...**

Fatigue is a best friend to stress. When you don't get enough sleep, it's hard to deal—you may feel tired, cranky, or you may have trouble thinking clearly. When you're overtired, a problem may seem much bigger than it actually is. You may have a hard time doing a school assignment that usually seems easy, you don't do your best in sports or any physical activity, or you may have an argument with your friends over something really stupid.

Sleep is a big deal! Getting the right amount of sleep is especially important for kids your age. Because your body (and mind) is changing and developing, it requires more sleep to re-charge for the next day. So don't resist, hit the hay!

8. **Keep a journal.**

If you're having one of those crazy days when nothing goes right, it's a good idea to write things down in a journal to get it off of your chest—like how you feel, what's going on in your life, and things you'd like to accomplish. You could even write down what you do when you're faced with a stressful situation, and then look back and think about how you handled it later. So, find a quiet spot, grab a notebook and pen, and start writing!

9. **Get it together.**

Too much to do but not enough time? Forgot your homework? Feeling overwhelmed or discombobulated? Being unprepared for school, practice, or other activities can make for a very stressful day!

Getting everything done can be a challenge, but all you have to do is plan a little and get organized.

10. **Lend a hand.**

Get involved in an activity that helps others. It's almost impossible to feel stressed out when you're helping someone else. It's also a great way to find out about yourself and the special qualities you never knew you had! Signing up for a service project is a good idea, but helping others is as easy as saying hello, holding a door, or volunteering to keep a neighbor's pet. If you want to get involved in a more organized volunteer program, try working at a local recreation center, or helping with an after school program. The feeling you will get from helping others is greater than you can imagine!

Most importantly, don't sweat the small stuff! Try to pick a few really important things and let the rest slide—getting worked up over every little thing will only increase your stress. So, toughen up and don't let stressful situations get to you! Remember, you're not alone—everyone has stresses in their lives—it's up to you to choose how to deal with them.

Chapter 60

Coping With A Disaster Or Traumatic Event

A traumatic event is a shocking, scary, or dangerous experience that affects someone emotionally. These situations may be natural, like a tornado or earthquake. They can also be caused by other people, like a car accident, crime, or terror attack.

Warning Signs

There are many different responses to potentially traumatic events. Most people have intense responses immediately following, and often for several weeks or even months after, a traumatic event. These responses can include:

- Feeling anxious, sad, or angry

- Trouble concentrating and sleeping

- Continually thinking about what happened

For most people, these are normal and expected responses and generally lessen with time. Healthy ways of coping in this time period include avoiding alcohol and other drugs, spending time with loved ones and trusted friends who are supportive, trying to maintain normal routines for meals, exercise, and sleep. In general, staying active is a good way to cope with stressful feelings.

About This Chapter: Text in this chapter begins with excerpts from "Coping With Traumatic Events," National Institute of Mental Health (NIMH), February 2017; Text under the heading "Trauma And Stress" is excerpted from "Helping Children And Adolescents Cope With Violence And Disasters," National Institute of Mental Health (NIMH), 2015; Text beginning with the heading "Common Reactions" is excerpted from "Coping With A Disaster Or Traumatic Event," Centers for Disease Control and Prevention (CDC), January 31, 2014.

However, in some cases, the stressful thoughts and feelings after a trauma continue for a long time and interfere with everyday life. For people who continue to feel the effects of the trauma, it is important to seek professional help. Some signs that an individual may need help include:

- Worrying a lot or feeling very anxious, sad, or fearful

- Crying often

- Having trouble thinking clearly

- Having frightening thoughts, reliving the experience

- Feeling angry

- Having nightmares or difficulty sleeping

- Avoiding places or people that bring back disturbing memories and responses

Physical responses to trauma may also mean that an individual needs help. Physical symptoms may include:

- Headaches

- Stomach pain and digestive issues

- Feeling tired

- Racing heart and sweating

- Being very jumpy and easily startled

Those who already had mental health problems or who have had traumatic experiences in the past, who are faced with ongoing stress, or who lack support from friends and family may be more likely to develop stronger symptoms and need additional help. Some people turn to alcohol or other drugs to cope with their symptoms. Although substance use can temporarily cover up symptoms, it can also make life more difficult.

Mental health problems can be treated. If you or someone you know needs help, talk with your healthcare provider.

Trauma And Stress

Some children will have prolonged mental health problems after a traumatic event. These may include grief, depression, anxiety, and post-traumatic stress disorder (PTSD). Some trauma survivors get better with some support. Others may need prolonged care from a mental health professional. If after a month in a safe environment children are not able to perform normal routines or new behavioral or emotional problems develop, then contact a health professional.

Factors influencing how someone may respond include:

- Being directly involved in the trauma, especially as a victim
- Severe and/or prolonged exposure to the event
- Personal history of prior trauma
- Family or personal history of mental illness and severe behavioral problems
- Limited social support; lack of caring family and friends
- Ongoing life stressors such as moving to a new home or new school, divorce, job change, or financial troubles

Some symptoms may require immediate attention. Contact a mental health professional if these symptoms occur:

- Flashbacks
- Racing heart and sweating
- Being easily startled
- Being emotionally numb
- Being very sad or depressed
- Thoughts or actions to end one's life

Common Reactions

For Preteens And Teenagers

Some preteens and teenagers respond with risky behaviors. This could include reckless driving, alcohol or drug use. Others may become afraid to leave home. They may cut way back on how much they hang out with their friends. They can feel overwhelmed by their intense emotions and yet be unable to talk about them. Those emotions may lead to increased friction, arguing and even fighting with siblings, parents/caregivers or other adults.

For Special-Needs Children

Children who are ventilator-dependent, or are confined to a wheelchair or bed, may have even more pronounced reactions to threatened or actual terrorism. The same is true for youth with other physical or mental limitations. They might display feelings like distress, worry or anger because they have less control over how they get around than other people. They may need extra verbal reassurance, or more explanations, hugs, comfort and other positive physical contact.

Not all children respond these ways. Some might have more severe, longer-lasting reactions that are influenced by the following factors:

- **Direct exposure to the disaster:** whether they were evacuated or saw people injured or dying would affect them, as would being injured themselves or feeling their own lives were threatened.

- **Loss:** the death or major injury of a family member, close friend or pet.

- **Ongoing stress from the effects of disaster:** this includes being away from home, losing contact with friends and neighbors and losing things that were important to them, like a favorite toy or access to a playground. Their lives are disrupted when they no longer have a usual meeting place or their routines and living conditions change.

- **A prior experience of trauma:** including having lived through or observed abuse or a major disaster.

What You Can Do To Help Others Cope With Disaster

- **Now:** Get informed; develop a family disaster plan; assemble disaster supplies kits; talk about your actions; think about how to handle stress; ask questions about things you don't understand; practice your plans; identify support networks in your community.

- **At the start of a disaster:** Listen to the authorities; show understanding; share facts with children; share plans to keep them safe.

- **During a disaster:** Calm fears that someone will be killed or injured; calm fears that children will be left alone or separated from their family; stay as connected as possible with kids and with others, as it provides care, support, and distraction.

- **After a disaster:** Calm fears that it will happen again.

How Can Children Learn To Cope?

Children base their reactions in part on what they see from the adults around them. When parents and caregivers deal with a disaster calmly and confidently, they can provide the best support for their children. The better prepared parents are, the more reassuring they are to others around them, especially children.

Self-care and preparation are critical for parents and caregivers. The more prepared, rested, and relaxed they are, the better they can respond to unexpected events and the more they can make decisions that will be in the best interest of those for whom they are responsible.

Children's reactions depend on their age and are affected by how close they are to an event, their level of exposure to it through TV, and how they see their parents and caregivers reacting.

Seeing repeated images of a disaster in the media can intensify people's distress. Early on, consider limiting the amount of exposure you want for yourself and your loved ones.

How Can Children With Disabilities Cope With Disaster And Traumatic Events?

When a disaster or traumatic event occurs, such as a natural disaster or violent act, whether accidental or intentional, it can be stressful for people of all ages. Children tend to react to disaster and traumatic events based on their past experiences and what they know of the current situation. Children with disabilities may require extra support from an adult to help them cope with disaster or traumatic events.

(Source: "Coping With Disaster And Traumatic Events," Centers for Disease Control and Prevention (CDC).)

Chapter 61

Playing Helps Kids Learn And Grow

What would childhood be without time to play? Play, it turns out, is essential to growing up healthy. Research shows that active, creative play benefits just about every aspect of child development.

Like adults, kids need exercise. Most children need at least an hour of physical activity every day. Regular exercise helps children

- Feel less stressed
- Feel better about themselves
- Feel more ready to learn in school
- Keep a healthy weight
- Build and keep healthy bones, muscles and joints
- Sleep better at night

As kids spend more time watching TV, they spend less time running and playing. Parents should limit TV, video game, and computer time. Parents can set a good example by being active themselves. Exercising together can be fun for everyone. Competitive sports can help kids stay fit. Walking or biking to school, dancing, bowling, and yoga are some other ways for kids to get exercise.

(Source: "Exercise For Children," National Institutes of Health (NIH).)

About This Chapter: This chapter includes text excerpted from "It's A Kid's Job," *NIH News in Health*, National Institutes of Health (NIH), June 2012. Reviewed July 2017.

How Playing Relates To Learning

"Play is behavior that looks as if it has no purpose," says National Institutes of Health (NIH) psychologist Dr. Stephen Suomi. "It looks like fun, but it actually prepares for a complex social world." Evidence suggests that play can help boost brain function, increase fitness, improve coordination and teach cooperation.

Suomi notes that all mammals—from mice to humans—engage in some sort of play. His research focuses on rhesus monkeys. While he's cautious about drawing parallels between monkeys and people, his studies offer some general insights into the benefits of play.

Active, vigorous social play during development helps to sculpt the monkey brain. The brain grows larger. Connections between brain areas may strengthen. Play also helps monkey youngsters learn how to fit into their social group, which may range from 30 to 200 monkeys in 3 or 4 extended families.

Both monkeys and humans live in highly complex social structures, says Suomi. "Through play, rhesus monkeys learn to negotiate, to deal with strangers, to lose gracefully, to stop before things get out of hand, and to follow rules," he says. These lessons prepare monkey youngsters for life after they leave their mothers.

Play may have similar effects in the human brain. Play can help lay a foundation for learning the skills we need for social interactions. If human youngsters lack playtime, says Dr. Roberta Golinkoff, an infant language expert at the University of Delaware, "social skills will likely suffer. You will lack the ability to inhibit impulses, to switch tasks easily and to play on your own." Play helps young children master their emotions and make their own decisions. It also teaches flexibility, motivation and confidence.

Kids don't need expensive toys to get a lot out of playtime. "Parents are children's most enriching plaything," says Golinkoff. Playing and talking to babies and children are vital for their language development. Golinkoff says that kids who talk with their parents tend to acquire a vocabulary that will later help them in school. "In those with parents who make a lot of demands, language is less well developed," she says. The key is not to take over the conversation, or you'll shut it down.

Advantages Of Playing

Unstructured, creative, physical play lets children burn calories and develops all kinds of strengths, such as learning how the world works. In free play, children choose the games, make the rules, learn to negotiate and release stress. Free play often involves fantasy. If children, say, want to learn about being a fireman, they can imagine and act out what a fireman does. And if something scary happens, free play can help defuse emotions by working them out.

"Sports are a kind of play, but it's not the kids calling the shots," says Golinkoff. It's important to engage in a variety of activities, including physical play, social play and solitary play. "The key is that in free play, kids are making the decisions," says Golinkoff. You can't learn to make decisions if you're always told what to do.

Dangers Of Eliminating Playing

Some experts fear that free play is becoming endangered. In the last 2 decades, children have lost an average of 8 hours of free play per week. As media screens draw kids indoors, hours of sitting raise the risk for obesity and related diseases. When it comes to video games and other media, parents should monitor content, especially violent content, and limit the amount of time children sit.

There's also been a national trend toward eliminating school recess. It's being pushed aside for academic study, including standardized test preparation. "Thousands of children have lost recess altogether," says child development expert Dr. Kathryn Hirsh-Pasek of Temple University. "Lack of recess has important consequences for young children who concentrate better when they come inside after a break from the schoolwork."

Many kids, especially those in low-income areas, lack access to safe places to play. This makes their school recess time even more precious. In response to these changes, some educators are now insisting that preschool and elementary school children have regular periods of active, free play with other children. The type of learning that happens during playtime is not always possible in the classroom. School recess is also important because of the growing number of obese children in the United States. Running around during recess can help kids stay at a healthy weight.

Play also may offer advantages within the classroom. In an NIH-funded study, Hirsh-Pasek, Golinkoff and their colleagues found a link between preschoolers' math skills and their ability to copy models of 2- and 3-dimensional building-block constructions. Play with building blocks—and block play alongside adults—can help build children's spatial skills so they can get an early start toward the later study of science, technology, engineering or math.

"In a way, a child is becoming a young scientist, checking out how the world works," says Hirsh-Pasek. "We never outgrow our need to play." Older children, including teens, also need to play and daydream, which helps their problem-solving and creative imagination. Adults, too, need their breaks, physical activity and social interaction.

At the NIH Clinical Center in Bethesda, Maryland, "Recreation therapy services are seen as essential to the patients' recovery," says Donna Gregory, chief of recreational therapy. She and her team tailor activities for both children and adults. Games can get patients moving, even for just minutes at a time, which improves their functioning.

Medical play helps children cope with invasive procedures. A 2-year-old can be distracted with blowing bubbles; older kids can place their teddy bear in the magnetic resonance imaging (MRI) machine or give their doll a shot before they themselves get an injection. It gives kids a sense of control and supports their understanding in an age-appropriate, meaningful way.

Without play and recreation, people can become isolated and depressed. "There's therapeutic value in helping patients maintain what's important to them," says Gregory. "When you are physically and socially active, it gives life meaning."

Chapter 62

Dealing With Divorce

> Divorce is the legal breakup of a marriage. Like every major life change, divorce is stressful. It affects finances, living arrangements, household jobs, schedules, and more. If the family includes children, they may be deeply affected.
>
> *(Source: "Divorce," National Institutes of Health (NIH).)*

The family is the first environment in which youth experience adult relationships. Family composition and adult behaviors—such as the presence of one or both parents and the quality and stability of their relationships—have long-lasting consequences for youth. Past research has consistently shown, for example, that children whose parents divorce are more likely to divorce themselves. Similarly, women born to unmarried mothers are more likely to have a nonmarital birth. Many factors related to family composition, such as income, parenting practices, and stress, could increase the likelihood that teens will have some of the same outcomes as their parents. In addition, the family structure in which children are raised is most familiar, and thus may seem a natural or normal choice when they later form their own families.

About This Chapter: Text in this chapter begins with excerpts from "Pathways To Adulthood And Marriage: Teenagers' Attitudes, Expectations, And Relationship Patterns," U.S. Department of Health and Human Services (HHS), October 2008. Reviewed July 2017; Text under the heading "Impact Of Parental Separation/Divorce" is excerpted from "Pathways To Adulthood And Marriage: Teenagers' Attitudes, Expectations, And Relationship Patterns. What Do Teens Think Of Their Parents' Relationships?" U.S. Department of Health and Human Services (HHS), October 1, 2008. Reviewed July 2017; Text under the heading "What To Do When Parents Divorce?" is excerpted from "Dealing With Loss And Grief," girlshealth.gov, Office on Women's Health (OWH), March 12, 2015; Text under the heading "Overcoming Parents' Divorce" is © 2017 Omnigraphics. Reviewed July 2017.

Impact Of Parental Separation/Divorce

The quality of their parents' relationship has important implications for youth. Past work has shown that parents' marital hostility is associated with behavioral and emotional problems in their children. Some work suggests that it is worse for children for their parents to remain in a conflict-ridden marriage than for their parents to divorce. The parents' relationship may also affect teens' views on marriage and relationships and the quality of their later relationships. For example, a recent study found that adolescent girls with more negative perceptions of the level of conflict in their parents' relationship had greater expectations of unhappiness and divorce in their own future marriages. Similarly, parental conflict after a divorce has been linked with less positive attitudes about marriage among adolescents.

Teens' perceptions of the parental relationship may not be the same as what the parents would say about their own relationship. The teens' perspective, however, is important because it indicates how they are experiencing that relationship. If teens think their parents are always fighting, for example, they are likely to feel stress and turmoil, regardless of whether the parents believe their fighting is frequent. Girls tend to view their parents' relationship more negatively than boys. Girls were more likely to view their parents' marriage as low quality and less likely to perceive the relationship as high quality.

What To Do When Parents Divorce

If your parents are getting divorced, it's normal to feel grief. So much of your life may be changing, and you may not have much control over what happens. You may feel angry, sad, lonely, scared, and lots of other emotions. All this can take time to heal.

There are many things you can do to feel better about a divorce. For starters, you can remember that divorce is never your fault.

Talk to your parents about how you're feeling. Tell them what would make the divorce easier on you. Get help from friends. You might also consider joining a support group for kids of divorcing parents. Your parents, school nurse, school counselor, or other adults can help you look for one. Also, see if you can think about any personal strengths that helped you in hard times before.

Ways To Feel Better

Everybody has the blues sometimes. The good news is that there are things you can do to feel better. Here are some tips to improve your mood:

- **Chill out.** Find a way to relax, such as taking a deep breath or taking a bath.

> - **Make a plan.** Life can feel out of control at times. Making a list of what you can do about a problem puts you back in charge.
> - **Focus on the positive.** Even in tough times, you likely have some good things going for you.
> - **Talk it out.** Talk to your friends, parents or guardians, teachers, counselors, or doctor about what you are feeling. They can help you sort through emotions and find solutions to problems.
>
> *(Source: "Feeling Sad," girlshealth.gov, Office on Women's Health (OWH).)*

Overcoming Parents' Divorce

Most teens face anxiety over the future when their parents' divorce. Will they change schools or move to a new house? Will they have to shuttle between parents? Will their financial circumstances change? To overcome that fear, teens should discuss their concerns with their parents at the right time when they are most receptive to listening.

Divorce is a life-changing event and causes significant stress for those involved. However, such events also allow individuals to realize their strengths and develop new skills to help them cope. Teens can seek the help of their close relatives, teachers, or counselors to help them in discovering their coping skills. They can find purpose in helping their younger siblings through this shared experience and can, as a result, develop special bonds with them.

Teens can overcome their grief over their parents' divorce by focusing on their own goals and ambitions. By doing so, teens can also reduce their stress and stay on course with their future. They can also take steps to improve their wellbeing by eating properly and exercising regularly. Teens can also distract themselves by concentrating on normal day-to-day activities when they feel depressed or upset.

References

1. Lyness D'Arcy, PhD. "Dealing With Divorce," The Nemours Foundation, January 2015.

2. Lyness D'Arcy, PhD. "Helping Your Child Through A Divorce," The Nemours Foundation, January 2015.

Chapter 63

Dealing With Grief

Grief is defined as the primarily emotional/affective process of reacting to the loss of a loved one through death. The focus is on the internal, intrapsychic process of the individual. Normal or common grief reactions may include components such as the following:

- Numbness and disbelief.

- Anxiety from the distress of separation.

- A process of mourning often accompanied by symptoms of depression.

- Eventual recovery.

Grief reactions can also be viewed as abnormal, traumatic, pathologic, or complicated. Although no consensus has been reached, diagnostic criteria for complicated grief have been proposed.

> **Feeling grief is normal. Every person has her own reactions to loss.** Here are some reactions you might have if you are grieving:
>
> - Strong emotions, such as sadness, anger, worry, or guilt
> - Few or no feelings, like you are emotionally numb
> - Crying spells or feeling like there's a lump in your throat

---

About This Chapter: Text in this chapter begins with excerpts from "Grief, Bereavement, And Coping With Loss (PDQ®)—Health Professional Version," National Cancer Institute (NCI), April 20, 2017; Text under the heading "Self-Care While Grieving" is excerpted from "Veterans Employment Toolkit—Dealing With Sadness Or Grief After A Loss," U.S. Department of Veterans Affairs (VA), September 2, 2015.

> - Physical reactions, such as having stomach aches or not sleeping
> - Spiritual reactions, like feeling disappointed in your religion or feeling even more connected to it
>
> Grief can go on for many months, but it should lessen over time. Everyone is different, but you should expect to feel at least a little better after a couple of months. If your grief doesn't get better over time, you may need the help of a therapist. Also, you should reach out for help without waiting if you have signs of depression. These include feeling worthless, having trouble functioning in your life, or thinking about hurting yourself.
>
> *(Source: "Dealing With Loss And Grief," girlshealth.gov, Office on Women's Health (OWH).)*

Types Of Grief Reactions

Many authors have proposed types of grief reactions. Research has focused on normal and complicated grief while specifying types of complicated grief and available empirical support with a focus on the characteristics of different types of dysfunction. Controversy over whether it is most accurate to think of grief as progressing in sequential stages (i.e., stage theories) continues. Most literature attempts to distinguish between normal grief and various forms of complicated grief such as chronic grief or absent/delayed/inhibited grief.

Bereavement research has tried to identify these patterns by reviewing available empirical support while also looking for evidence that these grief reactions are unique and not simply forms of major depression, anxiety, or posttraumatic stress.

Anticipatory Grief

Anticipatory grief refers to a grief reaction that occurs in anticipation of an impending loss. Anticipatory grief is the subject of considerable concern and controversy.

The term anticipatory grief is most often used when discussing the families of dying persons, although dying individuals themselves can experience anticipatory grief. Anticipatory grief includes many of the same symptoms of grief after a loss. Anticipatory grief has been defined as "the total set of cognitive, affective, cultural, and social reactions to expected death felt by the patient and family."

The following aspects of anticipatory grief have been identified among survivors:

- Depression.

- Heightened concern for the dying person.

- Rehearsal of the death.

- Attempts to adjust to the consequences of the death.

Normal Or Common Grief

In general, normal or common grief reactions are marked by a gradual movement toward an acceptance of the loss and, although daily functioning can be very difficult, managing to continue with basic daily activities. Normal grief usually includes some common emotional reactions that include emotional numbness, shock, disbelief, and/or denial often occurring immediately after the death, particularly if the death is unexpected. Much emotional distress is focused on the anxiety of separation from the loved one, which often results in yearning, searching, preoccupation with the loved one, and frequent intrusive images of death.

Over time, most bereaved people will experience symptoms less frequently, with briefer duration, or with less intensity. Although there is no clear agreement on any specific time period needed for recovery, most bereaved persons experiencing normal grief will note a lessening of symptoms at anywhere from 6 months through 2 years postloss. Normal or common grief appears to occur in 50 percent to 85 percent of persons following a loss, is time-limited, begins soon after a loss, and largely resolves within the first year or two.

Stage Models Of Normal Grief

A number of theoretically derived stage models of normal grief have been proposed. Most models hypothesize a normal grief process differentiated from various types of complicated grief. Some models have organized the variety of grief-related symptoms into phases or stages, suggesting that grief is a process marked by a series of phases, with each phase consisting of predominant characteristics. One well-known stage model, focusing on the responses of terminally ill patients to awareness of their own deaths, identified the stages of denial, anger, bargaining, depression, and acceptance. Although widely used, this model has received little empirical support.

A more recent stage model of normal grief organizes psychological responses into four stages: numbness-disbelief, separation distress, depression-mourning, and recovery. Although presented as a stage model, this model explains "it is important to emphasize that the idea that grief unfolds inexorably in regular phases is an oversimplification of the highly complex personal waxing and waning of the emotional process." Bereavement researchers have found empirical support for this four-stage model, although other researchers have questioned these findings.

357

Patterns Of Complicated Grief

Since the time of Sigmund Freud, many authors have proposed various patterns of pathologic or complicated grief. Some proposed patterns come from extensive clinical observation supported by various theories (e.g., psychodynamic defense mechanisms and personality traits associated with patterns of attachment).

These patterns are described in comparison to normal grief and highlight variations from the normal pattern. They include descriptive labels such as the following:

- **Inhibited or absent grief**: A pattern in which persons show little evidence of the expected separation distress, seeking, yearning, or other characteristics of normal grief.

- **Delayed grief**: A pattern in which symptoms of distress, seeking, yearning, etc., occur at a much later time than is typical.

- **Chronic grief**: A pattern emphasizing prolonged duration of grief symptoms.

- **Distorted grief**: A pattern characterized by extremely intense or atypical symptoms.

Prolonged Or Complicated Grief As A Mental Disorder

The *Diagnostic and Statistical Manual for Mental Disorders, Fourth Edition*, Text Revision (DSM-IV-TR) includes bereavement as a diagnosable code to be used when bereavement is a focus of clinical attention following the death of a loved one. In current form it does not consist of formal diagnostic criteria and is generally considered a normal reaction to loss via death. In an attempt to clearly distinguish between normal grief and complicated grief, a consensus conference has developed diagnostic criteria for a mental disorder referred to as prolonged grief disorder, proposing that it be included in the next revision of the DSM.

Following are the proposed diagnostic criteria for complicated grief:

- **Criterion A**: Person has experienced the death of a significant other, and response involves three of the four following symptoms, experienced at least daily or to a marked degree:

  - Intrusive thoughts about the deceased.

  - Yearning for the deceased.

  - Searching for the deceased.

  - Excessive loneliness since the death.

- **Criterion B**: In response to the death, four of the eight following symptoms are experienced at least daily or to a marked degree:

  - Purposelessness or feelings of futility about the future.

  - Subjective sense of numbness, detachment, or absence of emotional responsiveness.

  - Difficulty acknowledging the death (e.g., disbelief).

  - Feeling that life is empty or meaningless.

  - Feeling that part of oneself has died.

  - Shattered worldview (e.g., lost sense of security, trust, control).

  - Assumption of symptoms or harmful behaviors of, or related to, the deceased person.

  - Excessive irritability, bitterness, or anger related to the death.

- **Criterion C**: The disturbance (symptoms listed) must endure for at least 6 months.

- **Criterion D**: The disturbance causes clinically significant impairment in social, occupational, or other important areas of functioning.

These criteria have not been formally adopted, and thus there is no formal diagnostic category for prolonged grief disorders in the DSM. However, these criteria help in specifying symptoms, the severity of symptoms, and how to distinguish complicated grief from normal grief.

Children And Grief

At one time, children were considered miniature adults, and their behaviors were expected to be modeled as such. Today, there is a greater awareness of developmental differences between childhood and other developmental stages in the human life cycle. Differences between the grieving process for children and the grieving process for adults are recognized. It is now believed that the real issue for grieving children is not whether they grieve, but how they exhibit their grief and mourning.

The primary difference between bereaved adults and bereaved children is that intense emotional and behavioral expressions are not continuous in children. A child's grief may appear more intermittent and briefer than that of an adult, but in fact a child's grief usually lasts longer.

The work of mourning in childhood needs to be addressed repeatedly at different developmental and chronological milestones. Because bereavement is a process that continues over time, children will revisit the loss repeatedly, especially during significant life events (e.g., going to camp, graduating from school, marrying, and experiencing the births of their own children). Children must complete the grieving process, eventually achieving resolution of grief.

Although the experience of loss is unique and highly individualized, several factors can influence a child's grief:

- Age

- Personality

- Stage of development

- Previous experiences with death

- Previous relationship with the deceased

- Environment

- Cause of death

- Patterns of interaction and communication within the family

- Stability of family life after the loss

- How the child's needs for sustained care are met

- Availability of opportunities to share and express feelings and memories

- Parental styles of coping with stress

- Availability of consistent relationships with other adults

Children do not react to loss in the same ways as adults and may not display their feelings as openly as adults do. In addition to verbal communication, grieving children may employ play, drama, art, school work, and stories. Bereaved children may not withdraw into preoccupation with thoughts of the deceased person; they often immerse themselves in activities (e.g., they may be sad one minute and then playing outside with friends the next). Families often incorrectly interpret this behavior to mean the child does not really understand or has already gotten over the death. Neither assumption may be true; children's minds protect them from thoughts and feelings that are too powerful for them to handle.

Grief reactions are intermittent because children cannot explore all their thoughts and feelings as rationally as adults can. Additionally, children often have difficulty articulating their feelings about grief. A grieving child's behavior may speak louder than any words he or she could speak. Strong feelings of anger and fear of abandonment or death may be evident in the behaviors of grieving children. Children often play death games as a way of working out their feelings and anxieties in a relatively safe setting. These games are familiar to the children and provide safe opportunities to express their feelings.

Self-Care While Grieving

Taking care of yourself can help you through the process of grieving. Here are some tips:

- **Let yourself grieve.**

  Take time to experience the feelings that come with the loss. Let emotions come and go. This emotional pain can be very hard, but it's a basic part of healing.

- **Talk about your experience.**

  People may not know what you're going through. Talk to people you trust, at work and home, and let them know how to support you. Find someone who will listen without judgment. This might be a family member or friend, a chaplain or other spiritual counselor, a therapist, a Veteran or a support group.

- **Keep busy.**

  Do purposeful work that is consistent with your values.

- **Exercise.**

  Any bit of exercise can help, even just going for a short walk. Make a plan to get some form of exercise daily.

- **Eat well.**

  During times of distress, your body needs good food more than ever. Good nutrition can help you feel better physically and emotionally.

- **Wait to make major decisions.**

  Loss often involves unwanted or unexpected changes. Think about taking time to grieve before making major changes, such as selling your home or changing jobs.

- **Record your thoughts in a journal.**

  If you like to write, journaling can help. But if you find you feel worse after journaling, then stop and try another way of getting out your feelings.

- **Take advantage of your spiritual or religious beliefs.**

  You may find it helpful to call upon your spiritual beliefs to cope with your loss. Prayer or services, for instance, may be helpful. You might consult with a chaplain or pastoral counselor.

- **Get professional help if needed.**

  If you find that, over a period of time, your grief continues to interfere with your ability to move forward with your life, consider seeking help.

- You likely have strategies that you have found helpful when you experienced a loss in the past. Utilize the strategies that work best for you.

Chapter 64

Getting Along With Family And Friends

Someone took your seat at lunch or pushed ahead of you in line. Your best friend wants you to let her cheat off your test paper. A guy in math class called you—something not so nice. Sometimes it seems like life is a sea of problems—and your ship is sinking. BAM! Body and Mind can help you handle the things that make you crazy. (Well, not all of them. You'll still have homework.)

In every situation, everyone sees things differently and wants to do things their way. And it's normal for people to believe they are right, which leads to disagreements. Problems are never fun—but they can help you to have a good discussion and you can work things out. Clearing the air will help you learn more about your friends, your family and even yourself. Solving problems in the right way also can help you get through them quickly and easily, and stop them from getting out of control, or even violent.

If sparks do start to fly, you have the power to put out the fire. The next time you have an issue on your hands, don't explode or let someone walk all over you. Instead, convince them to try the BAM! plan with you.

Iron Out Your Issues

No plan will magically solve every problem or situation, but here are some ideas that have worked like a charm for other people.

About This Chapter: Text in this chapter begins with excerpts from "BAM! Guide To Getting Along," Centers for Disease Control and Prevention (CDC), May 9, 2015; Text beginning with the heading "Getting Along With Parents And Guardians" is excerpted from "Parents, Stepparents, Grandparents, And Guardians," girlshealth.gov, Office on Women's Health (OWH), September 16, 2015.

Take a moment.

Stepping back from the whole mess gives everyone a chance to cool down and think. When you're having a problem with someone, first take some time to understand your own thoughts and feelings. What's really the issue? For example, do you feel like you're not getting enough respect? What do you want? Why?

Next, find a time to work out the problem with the other person. Pick a quiet place where it's easy to talk. Make sure to give yourself enough time. (Out by the school buses 15 minutes before soccer practice probably isn't a good choice!)

Set the tone.

The "tone" is the mood of the talk. When you wake up in a bad mood, it can spoil the whole day, right? You want to make sure that your talk at least starts off with a good mood. Just saying "Let's work this out" can make a huge difference!

Agree on the problem.

Take turns telling your sides of the story. You can't solve a problem if you don't really understand everything that's going on.

When it's your turn, see how calm you can be. Speak softly, slowly, and firmly. No threats (like "If you don't shut up, I'll..."), because they can raise the problem to a whole new level-a bad one. No need to get all excited or mad!

Try giving your point of view this way: "I feel _____(angry, sad, or upset) when you_____ (take my stuff without permission, call me a name, or leave me out) because___(you should ask first, it hurts my feelings, or makes me feel lonely)." This really works to get people to listen, because they don't feel like you're judging them. Check out the difference. You could say "You're always late to pick me up!" or "I feel embarrassed when you pick me up late because all of my friends leave right on time and it seems like no one remembered me." You can also try just stating the facts. Instead of saying "You're a thief!" try "Maybe you picked up my shirt by mistake."

When it's the other person's turn, let them explain. Listen. Don't interrupt. Try to understand where they're coming from. Show that you hear them. When people aren't getting along, each person is part of the problem—but most of us tend to blame the other person. When you've done something wrong, be ready to say you're sorry.

The goal is to decide together what the real issues are. Do not pass "Go" until you do that. It's huge!

Think of solutions.

Take turns coming up with ways to solve the problem. Get creative. Usually, there are lots possible solutions. Next, talk about the good and bad points of each one.

Break The Anger Chain

Cool Rules

Ever notice how quickly people get angry? It seems like people can go from totally happy to totally ticked off in no time at all. In fact, the feeling of anger is actually a series of reactions that happen in just 1/30th of a second.

The amazing thing about anger is that it's not a basic emotion like, say, happiness. It is actually a secondary emotion and it is supposed to help keep you safe and protect you from danger—the ole' fight or flight thing! But if it gets out of hand or if you try to ignore it, it can lead to some serious issues. Here's how to break the chain.

Here is a simple way to remember how to deal with anger:

Stop it at the first spark.

Lots of things can trigger anger, like losing a soccer game, having to deal with your bossy little sister, or your computer crashing when you're in the middle of IM'ing your pals or writing a school paper. The important thing is to figure out what is really making you angry. Is it the same thing every time or do different things bring you to the boiling point? If it is always the same situation, person, or thing, try to avoid it. And if you can't avoid them (cuz' you know your little sister isn't going anywhere), think of different ways you can keep from getting angry. Instead of hurling the computer out the window, think about how you avoid it crashing to begin with, like not having your email and a game going at the same time. If losing the soccer game has got your goat, use your anger as motivation to improve your skills.

Hey, man! What's it all mean

So, snaps for figuring out how to spot the things you know make you angry. But, your little sister is still driving you nuts. Since she's staying put, you've got to figure out a way to handle your anger that won't make things worse. This brings us to the second link in the chain. To avoid it, all you need to do is try to look at things from her point of view—you're older and she wants to hang with you because she thinks you're cool. With that in mind, it's easier to keep your cool. Spend some time just with her so that she won't need to stalk you when all your friends are over. You might even find out that she's not half bad. By changing the way you deal with her and understanding her point of view, you can break the anger chain before you even notice you're mad!

Blood's a boilin

Well, ok, but your still furious. You've tried to change your reactions to the things that you know make you crazy, you're busy looking at everything from everyone else's point of view, but you can still feel your temperature is rising. Well, that's you're body responding to your feelings. You get hot and your muscles might start to tighten and you start breathing harder. Don't let it get the best of you—there are things you can do to stay in control. Take some deep breaths, focus on relaxing your muscles, and s-l-o-w down!

Talkin' to yourself?

The next link in the chain comes when you catch yourself thinking or saying something in reaction to what's happening to make you mad. We've all done it—we think things like "He's so stupid" or say to a friend "You're always so mean!" before we can stop ourselves. If you catch yourself doing this, take a minute to think. Try to remember that your dealing with a person who may not know how you feel. Stay calm. Lashing back won't get you anywhere. So try to talk to your friend, let him know he hurt your feelings, and then try to move on.

What you've got to do with it

The way you feel in a situation depends on your background—you may be used to people keeping their feelings in and not talking about them, or you may be used to people exploding and yelling when they are angry. Neither of these reactions is necessarily good. People who bottle up their feelings can end up exploding later, or become depressed. People who vent and yell just tend to keep the anger cycle in motion. The trick is to deal with your anger so that you can learn how to not get riled up in the first place. Try these suggestions to help you stay calm, cool, and collected.

- Go for a walk

- Write down your feelings on a piece of paper, then tear it up and throw it away

- Face the mirror and practice talking to the person that you are mad at

That's the way the story ends…

Isn't it amazing how many things come in between the first spark and being really mad? The whole chain happens so fast because we train ourselves to react in a certain way without even knowing we're doing it. But if you learn to recognize the steps in between, you can break the chain before you lose your cool. No matter how hard you try, you won't be able to avoid getting angry in every situation. You just have to decide the best way to respond. Anger doesn't have to be negative—if you handle it the right way it can actually clue you in to dangerous situations and make you a stronger person.

Getting Along With Parents And Guardians

- As you get older, your relationship with your parents or guardians changes. You may want more privacy or independence, for example. That's natural, but you can still stay connected.

- Making time to talk can help strengthen your connections. You might just talk about simple, everyday things or talk while doing something fun together. Being in the habit of talking about small things may make it easier to talk about harder subjects.

- If you want to share how you feel about something, it can be easier if you use "I statements." That means you say things like "I feel…" instead of criticizing the other person. Also, if you want something, try to ask politely. (Making demands is not very polite—or very effective.)

- If you need to raise a tough topic, keep in mind that your parents or guardians were young once, too. They may have faced very similar issues. Plus, they probably will appreciate your honesty and bravery in coming to them.

- If you don't like your family's rules, ask if you can discuss them. Sometimes, parents are willing to change certain rules, especially if you show you can be responsible.

Tips For Handling Fights With Parents

- **Talk about the rules.** Ask the reasons behind a rule so you can understand it. Consider sharing how a rule makes you feel. Ask if your parents or guardians will consider your ideas about what the rules should be.

- **Follow the rules.** Keep to your curfew if you have one. Call if you're going to be late, so your parents or guardians don't worry. If you follow the rules, your parents or guardians may be more likely to discuss them. If you don't follow the rules, you'll likely just get in trouble.

- **Pick your battles.** Cleaning your room is no fun, but it's most likely not worth fighting about.

- **Spend time with your family.** Some teens fight with their parents or guardians over how much time they spend with friends. Talk it over, and make some special family time. You might go for a walk or have dinner together.

- **Try to stay calm.** Don't yell or stomp your feet when your parents or guardians say no. If you listen and speak calmly, you may show them that you are growing up.

- **After an argument, think about what happened.** Consider your part in the problem, and apologize. Talk about how you might prevent similar fights in the future.

Getting Along With Stepparents

A new stepparent can bring up lots of feelings. Even if you like your stepparent, you may feel sad, worried, or upset at times.

Here are some tips that can help:

- **Accept your feelings.** It's natural to have feelings like confusion, anger, and guilt when a parent remarries. Don't worry that there's something wrong with you if you have any (or all) of these feelings!

- **Sort through your feelings.** Keeping a journal might help. Friends who have gone through a similar situation may also be able to offer tips.

- **Talk honestly.** If you don't like any new rules or situations, ask calmly and respectfully about changing them.

- **Get support from your parent or another trusted adult.** Adults who care about you really want to help. If it seems too hard to turn to a family member, talk to another adult you trust. If you are struggling, a mental health professional like a school counselor can help.

- **Try to spend time with your stepparent.** This new person is going to be around, and chances are you will be happier if you can find his or her more positive sides.

Keep in mind that with patience—and some hard work—lots of stepfamilies end up feeling very close.

Chapter 65

Running Away Doesn't Solve Problems

Many teens think about running away from home at some point. If you are thinking about running away, you can get help, and you can learn more about life as a runaway.

If You Are Thinking About Running Away

Running away comes with a lot of possible problems. Teens who run away face a high risk of living on the streets, going hungry, and other serious worries. If you are thinking about running away, here are a few questions to ask yourself:

- Are there things you can do to improve the situation at home?
- What would make it okay to stay at home?
- Where will you stay if you leave?
- What will you do for money and food?
- Is running away safe?
- Who can you count on for help?
- Are you being realistic about what life would be like if you leave?
- What are your other options?
- If you end up in trouble, who will you call?
- If you want to go home, what will happen?

About This Chapter: This chapter includes text excerpted from "Running Away," girlshealth.gov, Office on Women's Health (OWH), January 7, 2015.

Signs That A Friend May Run Away

Signs that someone may be thinking about running away include:

- Changes in eating or sleeping habits

- Dramatic mood swings

- Problems with school attendance or behavior

- Starting to carry lots of money and possibly even asking you to hold some of it

- Giving away clothing and other valuable items

- Saying things like, "Do you think anyone would miss me if I leave home?"

Running away is serious. Some of the items above could be signs of other problems, such as depression. If you think a friend may be depressed or having other problems, ask. You could really help someone. If a problem is too much for you to handle alone, make sure to talk to an adult.

How To Help A Friend Who Is Thinking About Running Away

You can be a great friend to someone who is thinking about running away. You can't solve the person's problems, but you can offer support. Below are some ways you can help.

Ask questions to help your friend think through running away.

Talk to your friend about life on the street. Being homeless can be extremely scary and dangerous. For example:

- Young people who are homeless are more likely to be victims of crime and sexual abuse.

- Around 1 out of 10 young people at runaway or homeless youth shelters have traded sex for food, a place to stay, or other things. Around 1 out of 3 young people who live on the streets have done this.

- Teens who run away have higher rates of depression, alcohol, and drug problems.

- One out of 4 young people who live on the street had a serious health problem in the past year.

- Girls who run away are more likely to get pregnant.

See if your friend can get help. Encourage your friend to talk to her or his parents. If that doesn't work, suggest that your friend talk to other relatives, a teacher, a school counselor, or another trusted adult.

See if your friend can stay with you for a couple of days. Things at your friend's house may calm down during that time. Or your friend may be able to find another place to stay if going home is not possible.

Why Do Teens Run Away?

The most common reason that teens run away is family problems. Family problems might include fights over things like money, grades, or strict rules.

Teens also may run away to try to escape worries like having problems with school, being bullied, coming out as gay, or dealing with an unplanned pregnancy. Alcohol or drugs also can play a role in teens' running away.

Often, teens may run away because of emotional, physical, or sexual abuse at home. If a friend is being abused, you can get help. Talk to your parents or another trusted adult, the police, local child protective services. Encourage your friend to reach out to a trusted adult like a teacher, counselor, neighbor, or clergy person. Offer to go along for support.

Running Away And Family Problems

Sometimes, girls want to leave home because of family problems. A girl may feel that her parents or other caregivers have unfair demands or rules. Or she may feel like they don't get her or don't take her seriously.

If you are thinking about running away because of family problems, see if you can work on your relationship with your parents or caregivers. Here are some tips you can try:

- Set aside some time to talk every day. You can even talk about just small things to start to connect better.

- Do things together, like running errands or watching a movie.

- Say what you think and need. Remember that adults can't read your mind.

- Have patience. Good communication takes time and effort.

- Work together to think up possible solutions to problems.

- Make a list of changes you want to see. Sometimes it's easier to write things down.

- Be willing to compromise. It's better to come away with part of what you want than to be stuck in a fight.

- Try to find a time and place with few distractions if you have something important to discuss.

- Use resources in your community when you need help working out family problems. Ask a teacher or school counselor for suggestions.

Talking To Your Parents About Emotional Problems

It takes courage to tell a parent or guardian that you are having trouble with your feelings. But adults can help you through tough times, and it's important to get the support you need.

When you're ready, try to find a time when you won't get interrupted. You may even need to schedule a time to talk. Try saying something like, "Mom and Dad, I have something I'd like to talk about. Can we sit and talk after dinner?"

If talking seems too hard, it might be easier to write your thoughts. A letter, an email, or even a text message can get the conversation going. Try something as simple as "I've been feeling anxious" or "I'm worried I might be depressed." Or you might just say, "I need your help."

Keep in mind that if your parents or you get upset, you can continue the conversation over time. If they ask a question about your feelings that you can't answer, you might say you'll think about it and will talk more later.

If you think you definitely can't talk to your parents or guardians, reach out to another trusted adult. This might be a school counselor, teacher, religious leader, school nurse, or doctor. Definitely don't give up. You deserve to feel better!

(Source: "Talking To Your Parents About Emotional Problems," girlshealth.gov, Office on Women's Health (OWH).)

Chapter 66

Suicide Prevention

Suicide is when people direct violence at themselves with the intent to end their lives, and they die as a result of their actions. Suicide is a leading cause of death in the United States. A suicide attempt is when people harm themselves with the intent to end their lives, but they do not die as a result of their actions. Many more people survive suicide attempts than die, but they often have serious injuries. However, a suicide attempt does not always result in a physical injury.

People who attempt suicide and survive may experience serious injuries, such as broken bones, brain damage, or organ failure. These injuries may have long-term effects on their health. People who survive suicide attempts may also have depression and other mental health problems. Suicide also affects the health of others and the community. When people die by suicide, their family and friends often experience shock, anger, guilt, and depression. The medical costs and lost wages associated with suicide also take their toll on the community.

Suicide is a serious public health problem that can have lasting harmful effects on individuals, families, and communities. While its causes are complex and determined by multiple factors, the goal of suicide prevention is simple: Reduce factors that increase risk (i.e., risk factors) and increase factors that promote resilience (i.e., protective factors). Ideally, prevention addresses all levels of influence: individual, relationship, community, and societal. Effective prevention strategies are needed to promote awareness of suicide and encourage a commitment to social change.

(Source: "Violence Prevention—Suicide," Centers for Disease Control and Prevention (CDC).)

Suicide In America[1]

Suicide does not discriminate. People of all genders, ages, and ethnicities can be at risk for suicide. But people most at risk tend to share certain characteristics. The main risk factors for suicide are:

About This Chapter: This chapter includes text excerpted from documents published by two public domain sources. Text under the headings marked 1 are excerpted from "Suicide In America: Frequently Asked Questions (2015)," National Institute of Mental Health (NIMH), April 2015; Text under the headings marked 2 are excerpted from "Feeling Suicidal," girlshealth.gov, Office on Women's Health (OWH), January 7, 2015.

- Depression, other mental disorders, or substance abuse disorder

- A prior suicide attempt

- Family history of a mental disorder or substance abuse

- Family history of suicide

- Family violence, including physical or sexual abuse

- Having guns or other firearms in the home

- Incarceration, being in prison or jail

- Being exposed to others' suicidal behavior, such as that of family members, peers, or media figures

The risk for suicidal behavior is complex. Research suggests that people who attempt suicide differ from others in many aspects of how they think, react to events, and make decisions. There are differences in aspects of memory, attention, planning, and emotion, for example. These differences often occur along with disorders like depression, substance use, anxiety, and psychosis. Sometimes suicidal behavior is triggered by events such as personal loss or violence. In order to be able to detect those at risk and prevent suicide, it is crucial that we understand the role of both long-term factors—such as experiences in childhood—and more immediate factors like mental health and recent life events. Researchers are also looking at how genes can either increase risk or make someone more resilient to loss and hardships.

Many people have some of these risk factors but do not attempt suicide. Suicide is not a normal response to stress. It is, however, a sign of extreme distress, not a harmless bid for attention.

What About Gender?[1]

Men are more likely to die by suicide than women, but women are more likely to attempt suicide. Men are more likely to use deadlier methods, such as firearms or suffocation. Women are more likely than men to attempt suicide by poisoning.

What About Children?[1]

Children and young people are at risk for suicide. Suicide is the second leading cause of death for young people ages 15 to 34.

Why Do Some Teens Think About Suicide?[2]

Some teens feel so terrible and overwhelmed that they think life will never get better. Some things that may cause these feelings include:

- The death of someone close

- Having depression or other mental health issues, such as an eating disorder, ADHD, or anxiety

- Having alcohol or drug problems

- Parents getting divorced

- Seeing a lot of anger and violence at home

- Having a hard time in school

- Being bullied

- Having problems with friends

- Experiencing a trauma like being raped or abused

- Being angry or heartbroken over a relationship break-up

- Feeling like you don't belong, either in your family or with friends

- Feeling rejected because of something about you, like being gay

- Having an ongoing illness or disability

- Feeling alone

- Feeling guilty or like a burden to other people

Also, teens sometimes may feel very bad for no one clear reason. If you are suffering, know that things definitely can get better. You can learn ways to handle your feelings. You can work toward a much brighter future.

Turning to others can help you through tough times. If you don't feel a strong connection to relatives or friends, try talking to a school counselor, teacher, doctor, or another adult you trust.

Every teen feels anxiety, sadness, and confusion at some point. The important thing to remember is that life can get much better. There is always help out there for you or a friend.

How Can Suicide Be Prevented?[1]

Effective suicide prevention is based on sound research. Programs that work take into account people's risk factors and promote interventions that are appropriate to specific groups of people. For example, research has shown that mental and substance abuse disorders are risk factors for suicide. Therefore, many programs focus on treating these disorders in addition to addressing suicide risk specifically.

Psychotherapy, or "talk therapy," can effectively reduce suicide risk. One type is called cognitive behavioral therapy (CBT). CBT can help people learn new ways of dealing with stressful experiences by training them to consider alternative actions when thoughts of suicide arise.

Another type of psychotherapy called dialectical behavior therapy (DBT) has been shown to reduce the rate of suicide among people with borderline personality disorder, a serious mental illness characterized by unstable moods, relationships, self-image, and behavior. A therapist trained in DBT helps a person recognize when his or her feelings or actions are disruptive or unhealthy, and teaches the skills needed to deal better with upsetting situations.

Medications may also help; promising medications and psychosocial treatments for suicidal people are being tested.

Still other research has found that many older adults and women who die by suicide saw their primary care providers in the year before death. Training doctors to recognize signs that a person may be considering suicide may help prevent even more suicides.

What Should I Do If Someone I Know Is Considering Suicide?[1]

If you know someone who is considering suicide, do not leave him or her alone. Try to get your loved one to seek immediate help from his or her doctor or the nearest hospital emergency room, or call 911. Remove any access he or she may have to firearms or other potential tools for suicide, including medications.

If You Are In Crisis[1]

Call the toll-free National Suicide Prevention Lifeline at 1-800-273-8255, available 24 hours a day, 7 days a week. The service is available to anyone. All calls are confidential.

What If Someone I Know Attempts Or Dies By Suicide?[2]

If someone you know attempts or dies by suicide, you may feel like it's your fault in some way. That's not true! You also may feel many different emotions, including anger, grief, or even emotional numbness. All of your feelings are okay. There is not a right or wrong way to feel.

If you are having trouble dealing with your feelings, talk to a trusted adult. You have suffered a terrible loss, but life can feel okay again. Reach out to people who care about you. Connecting is so important at this tough time.

Part Eight
If You Need More Information

Chapter 67

Additional Resources For Mental Health And Mental Illness

Other Teen Health Books from Omnigraphics

Abuse and Violence Information For Teens, Second Edition

Health Tips About The Causes And Consequences Of Abusive And Violent Behavior Including Facts About The Types Of Abuse And Violence, The Warning Signs Of Abusive And Violent Behavior, Health Concerns Of Victims, And Getting Help And Staying Safe

Alcohol Information For Teens, Fourth Edition

Health Tips About Alcohol Use, Abuse, And Dependence Including Facts About Alcohol's Effects On Mental And Physical Health, The Consequences Of Underage Drinking, And Understanding Alcoholic Family Members

Drug Information for Teens, Fourth Edition

Health Tips About The Physical And Mental Effects Of Substance Abuse Including Information About Alcohol, Tobacco, Marijuana, E-Cigarettes, Cocaine, Prescription And Over-The-Counter Drugs, Club Drugs, Hallucinogens, Heroin, Stimulants, Opiates, Steroids, And More

Eating Disorders Information For Teens, Fourth Edition

Health Tips About Anorexia, Bulimia, Binge Eating, And Body Image Disorders Including Information About Risk Factors, Prevention, Diagnosis, Treatment, Health Consequences, And Other Related Issues

About This Chapter: The mobile apps listed in this chapter were compiled from several sources deemed reliable. Inclusion does not constitute endorsement, and there is no implication associated with omission. All Website information was verified and updated in July 2017.

Learning Disabilities Information For Teens, Second Edition

Health Tips About Academic Skills Disorders And Other Disabilities That Affect Learning Including Information About Common Signs Of Learning Disabilities, School Issues, Learning To Live With A Learning Disability, And Other Related Issues

Suicide Information For Teens, Third Edition

Health Tips About Suicide Causes And Prevention Including Facts About Depression, Risk Factors, Getting Help, Survivor Support, And More

Mobile Apps For Mental Health

Anxiety

At Ease Anxiety & Worry Relief

This app is designed to relieve anxiety and worry by combining voice-guided breathing meditations, mental exercises and journaling.
Website: www.meditationoasis.com/at-ease-anxiety-worry-relief-app

Beat Panic

This app contains a series of flashcards designed in soothing colors and texts that assist in overcoming the panic attack in a gentle calm manner.
Website: https://itunes.apple.com/gb/app/beat-panic/id452656397?mt=8

Breathe to Relax

This is portable stress management tool that provides detailed information on the effects of stress on the body and instructions and practice to help users learn the stress management skill called diaphragmatic breathing.
Website: www.t2health.dcoe.mil/apps/breathe2relax

iCBT

This app is designed to help its users to manage stress and anxiety.
Website: https://itunes.apple.com/us/app/icbt/id355021834?mt=8

MindShift

This app helps users to relax, develop more helpful ways of thinking, and identify active steps that will help to take charge of anxiety. It also includes strategies to deal with everyday anxiety.
Website: www.anxietybc.com/resources/mindshift-app

Pacifica

This app contains tools for stress and anxiety alongside a supportive community developed based on cognitive behavioral therapy and meditation.
Website: www.thinkpacifica.com

Panic Relief

This app guides a person through panic attacks and helps to overcome fear.
Website: www.cognitivetherapyapp.com

Self-Help Anxiety Management

This app is designed to help its users understand and manage anxiety.
Website: www.sam-app.org.uk

Worry Box—Anxiety Self-Help

This app is to learn to control worry and get relief from anxiety.
Website: www.excelatlife.com/apps.htm

Depression

Depression CBT Self-Help Guide

This app is developed to offer self-help for depression.
Website: www.excelatlife.com/apps.htm#depressionapp

Mood Sentry

This app designed to help porting of multiple computer based tools used to manage depression to a mobile platform.
Website: www.moodsentry.com

MoodMission

This is an evidence-based app designed to empower people to overcome low moods and anxiety by discovering new and better ways of coping.
Website: www.moodmission.com/app

Mood Charting

MoodPanda

This apps is designed to help people track their moods and to get anonymous support.
Website: www.moodpanda.com

My Life My Voice

This mood journal offers a simple solution for tracking thoughts, feelings, and moods.
Website: www.yourlifeyourvoice.org/Pages/mobile-app.aspx

Posttraumatic Stress Disorder (PTSD)

Bust PTSD

This app is designed to help people who have experienced posttraumatic stress disorder or living with PTSD symptoms.
Website: www.cceipar.com/#section-app

Suicide Prevention

ASK & Prevent Suicide

This app helps to learn the warning signs and how to ask if someone is considering suicide.
Website: www.mhatexas.org/find-help

HELP Prevent Suicide

This app provides easy access to crisis intervention resources, including a list of warning signs, steps on how to talk with someone in crisis, and information on national resources.
Website: www.app.staplegun.us/help_prevent_suicide

Lifebuoy

Lifebuoy is an interactive, self-help promoting app designed to assist suicide survivors as they normalize their lives after recent attempt.
Website: www.itunes.apple.com/us/app/lifebuoy-suicide-prevention/id686973252

R U Suicidal?

This is a video-based, interactive self-help tool for anyone having thoughts about suicide.
Website: www.psychappsint.com

Suicide Lifeguard

This app is intended for anyone concerned that someone they know may be thinking of suicide. It provides information on warning signs of suicide, suicidal thoughts and/or intentions, and how to respond to them.
Website: www.mimhtraining.com/suicide-lifeguard

Suicide Safety Plan

This app provides six evidence-based tools to aid against clinical depression and negative moods on a large scale.
Website: www.moodtools.org

Chapter 68

Crisis Help And Hotlines

Alcohol And Drugs

Al-Anon/Alateen
Toll-Free: 888-425-2666
Phone: 757-563-1600
Website: www.al-anon.alateen.org
E-mail: wso@al-anon.org

Narconon
Toll-Free: 800-775-8750
Website: www.narconon.org

National Alcohol and Substance Abuse Information Center (NASAIC)
Toll-Free: 800-784-6776
Website: www.addictioncareoptions.com

National Institute On Drug Abuse (NIDA) For Teens
Toll-Free: 800-662-HELP (800-662-4357)
Website: www.teens.drugabuse.gov

About This Chapter: Resources in this chapter were compiled from several sources deemed reliable; all contact information was verified and updated in July 2017.

Bullying And Cyberbullying

No More Bullying, Live Empowered (NOBLE)
Phone: 317-375-2700
Website: www.mynoblelife.org

Thursday's Child National Youth Advocacy Hotline
Toll-Free: 800-USA-KIDS (800-872-5437)
Phone: 818-831-1234
Website: www.thursdayschild.org

The Trevor Project
Crisis intervention for lesbian, gay, bisexual, transgender, and questioning (LGBTQ)
Toll-Free: 866-488-7386
Phone: 202-304-1200 or text TREVOR (Monday through Friday between: 3pm–10pm EST/12pm–7pm PT)
Website: www.thetrevorproject.org

Depression

Crisis Call Center
Toll-Free: 800-273-TALK (800-273-8255) or text ANSWER to 839863
Phone: 775-784-8090
Website: www.crisiscallcenter.org
E-mail: info@crisiscallcenter.org

National Hopeline Network
Toll-Free: 800-SUICIDE (800-784-2433) / Toll-Free: 800-442-HOPE (800-442-4673)
Website: www.hopeline.com

Eating Disorders

National Association of Anorexia Nervosa and Associated Disorders (ANAD)
Phone: 630-577-1330
Website: www.anad.org
E-mail: hello@anad.org

National Eating Disorders Association (NEDA)
Toll-Free: 800-931-2237 (9 a.m. to 9 p.m. EST, Monday through Thursday; until 5 p.m. on Friday)
Website: www.nationaleatingdisorders.org

Grief And Loss

Tragedy Assistance Program for Survivors (TAPS)
Toll-Free: 800-959-TAPS (800-959-8277)
Phone: 202-588-8277
Website: www.taps.org

Homelessness And Runaways

Boys Town National Hotline
Serving all at-risk teens and children
Toll-Free: 800-448-3000
Website: www.boystown.org
E-mail: helpkids@boystown.org

National Runaway Safeline
Toll-Free: 800-RUNAWAY (800-786-2929)
Website: www.1800runaway.org
E-mail: info@1800runaway.org

National Safe Place
Toll-Free: 888-290-7233 or text SAFE and your current location (address/city/state) to 69866
Website: www.nationalsafeplace.org
E-mail: info@nationalsafeplace.org

Mental Health

National Alliance on Mental Illness (NAMI) Information Helpline
Toll-Free: 800-950-NAMI (800-950-6264; 10 a.m.–6 p.m. EST, Monday through Friday)
Website: www.nami.org
E-mail: info@nami.org

National Institute of Mental Health (NIMH) Information Center
Toll-Free: 866-615-6464 (8.30 a.m. to 5 p.m. EST, Monday through Friday)
Toll-Free TTY: 866-415-8051
Website: www.nimh.nih.gov
E-mail: nimhinfo@nih.gov

Mental Health America (MHA)
Formerly known as the National Mental Health Association (NMHA)
Toll-Free: 800-273-TALK (800-273-8255) or text MHA to 741741 at the Crisis Text Line
Phone: 703-684-7722
Website: www.mentalhealthamerica.net

Rape, Sexual Violence, And Domestic Violence

Childhelp National Child Abuse Hotline
Toll-Free: 800-4-A-CHILD (800-422-4453)
Phone: 480-922-8212
Website: www.childhelp.org

CyberTipline
National Center for Missing & Exploited Children (NCMEC)
Toll-Free: 800-THE-LOST (1-800-843-5678)
Phone: 703-224-2150
Website: www.missingkids.org

loveisrespect, National Teen Dating Abuse Helpline
Toll-Free: 866-331-9474 or text LOVEIS to 22522
Toll-Free TTY: 866-331-8453
Website: www.loveisrespect.org

The National Domestic Violence Hotline
Toll-Free: 800-799-SAFE (800-799-7233)
Toll-Free TTY: 800-787-3224
Phone: 512-453-8117
Website: www.thehotline.org

Rape, Abuse, and Incest National Network (RAINN)
Toll-Free: 800-656-HOPE (800-656-4673)
Website: www.rainn.org

Safe Horizon's Rape, Sexual Assault, and Incest Hotline
Toll-Free: 800-621-HOPE (800-6214673; Domestic Violence Hotline) / Toll-Free: 866-689-HELP (866-689-4357; Crime Victims Hotline)
Toll-Free TDD: 866-604-5350 (for all hotlines)
Phone: 212-227-3000 (Rape, Sexual Assault, and Incest Hotline)
Website: www.safehorizon.org
E-mail: help@safehorizon.org

SPEAK UP!
Toll-Free: 866-SPEAK-UP (866-773-2587)
Website: www.speakup.com

Sexuality And Sexual Health

Lesbian, Gay, Bisexual and Transgender (LGBT) National Youth Talkline
Toll-Free: 800-246-PRIDE (800-246-7743) Monday through Friday from 1pm to 9pm, Pacific Time
Website: www.glnh.org
E-mail: help@LGBThotline.org

Suicide

Kristin Brooks Hope Center (KBHC)
Toll-Free: 800-SUICIDE (800-784-2433) / Toll-Free: 800-442-HOPE (800-442-4673)
Website: www.hopeline.com
E-mail: info@imalive.org

National Suicide Prevention Lifeline
Toll-Free: 800-273-TALK (800-273-8255)
Toll-Free TTY: 800-799-4TTY (800-799-4889)
Website: www.suicidepreventionlifeline.org

Chapter 69

Directory Of Mental Health Organizations

National Mental Health Resources

Al-Anon Family Group Headquarters

1600 Corporate Landing Pkwy
Virginia Beach, VA 23454-5617
Phone: 757-563-1600
Fax: 757-563-1655
Website: www.al-anon.alateen.org
E-mail: wso@al-anon.org

American Academy of Child and Adolescent Psychiatry

3615 Wisconsin Ave. N.W.
Washington, DC 20016-3007
Phone: 202-966-7300
Fax: 202-464-0131
Website: www.aacap.org
E-mail: clinical@aacap.org

American Art Therapy Association

4875 Eisenhower Ave., Ste. 240
Alexandria, VA 22304
Toll-Free: 888-290-0878
Phone: 703-548-5860
Fax: 703-783-8468
Website: www.arttherapy.org
E-mail: info@arttherapy.org

American Association for Marriage and Family Therapy

112 S. Alfred St.
Alexandria, VA 22314-3061
Phone: 703-838-9808
Fax: 703-838-9805
Website: www.aamft.org
E-mail: central@aamft.org

About This Chapter: Resources in this chapter were compiled from several sources deemed reliable; all contact information was verified and updated in July 2017.

American Association of Suicidology

5221 Wisconsin Ave. N.W.
Washington, DC 20015
Phone: 202-237-2280
Fax: 202-237-2282
Website: www.suicidology.org
E-mail: info@suicidology.org

American Counseling Association

6101 Stevenson Ave.
Alexandria, VA 22304
Toll-Free: 800-347-6647
Phone: 703-823-9800
TDD: 703-823-6862
Toll-Free Fax: 800-473-2329
Fax: 703-823-0252
Website: www.counseling.org
E-mail: membership@counseling.org

American Foundation for Suicide Prevention

120 Wall St. 29th Fl.
New York, NY 10005
Toll-Free: 888-333-AFSP (888-333-2377)
Phone: 212-363-3500
Fax: 212-363-6237
Website: www.afsp.org
E-mail: inquiry@afsp.org

American Psychiatric Association

1000 Wilson Blvd.
Ste. 1825
Arlington, VA 22209-3901
Toll-Free: 888-35-PSYCH (888-357-7924)
Phone: 703-907-7300
Website: www.psychiatry.org
E-mail: apa@psych.org

American Psychological Association

750 First St. N.E.
Washington, DC 20002-4242
Toll-Free: 800-374-2721
Phone: 202-336-5500
TDD/TTY: 202-336-6123
Website: www.apa.org
E-mail: public.affairs@apa.org

American Psychotherapy Association

2750 E. Sunshine St.
Springfield, MO 65804
Toll-Free: 800-205-9165
Phone: 417-823-0173
Fax: 417-823-9959
Website: www.americanpsychotherapy.com
E-mail: cao@americanpsychotherapy.com

Anxiety Disorders Association of America

8701 Georgia Ave.
Ste. 412
Silver Spring, MD 20910
Phone: 240-485-1001
Fax: 240-485-1035
Website: www.adaa.org
E-mail: information@adaa.org

Association for Applied Psychophysiology and Biofeedback

10200 W. 44th Ave.
Ste. 304
Wheat Ridge, CO 80033
Toll-Free: 800-477-8892
Phone: 303-422-8436
Website: www.aapb.org
E-mail: info@aapb.org

Association for Behavioral and Cognitive Therapies

305 Seventh Ave.
16th Fl.
New York, NY 10001
Phone: 212-647-1890
Fax: 212-647-1865
Website: www.abct.org
E-mail: membership@abct.org

Beyond Blue Ltd.

Level 2
290 Burwood Rd.
Hawthorn Vic 3122
Australia
Phone: 03-9810 6100
Fax: 03-9810-6111
Website: www.beyondblue.org.au

Brain and Behavior Research Foundation

90 Park Ave.
16th Fl.
New York, NY 10016
Toll-Free: 800-829-8289
Phone: 646-681-4888
Website: www.bbrfoundation.org
E-mail: info@bbrfoundation.org

Brain Injury Association of America

1608 Spring Hill Rd.
Ste. 110
Vienna, VA 22182
Toll-Free: 800-444-6443
Phone: 703-761-0750
Fax: 703-761-0755
Website: www.biausa.org
E-mail: info@biausa.org

Caring.com

2600 S. El Camino Real, Ste. 300
San Mateo, CA 94403
Toll-Free: 800-973-1540.
Phone: 650-312-7100
Website: www.caring.com

Depressed Anonymous

P.O. Box 17414
Louisville, KY 40217
Website: www.depressedanon.com
E-mail: depanon@netpenny.net

Depression and Bipolar Support Alliance

55 E. Jackson Blvd., Ste. 490
Chicago, IL 60604
Toll-Free: 800-826-3632
Fax: 312-642-7243
Website: www.dbsalliance.org

Eating Disorder Referral and Information Center

Website: www.edreferral.com

Families for Depression Awareness

391 Totten Pond Rd.
Ste. 101
Waltham, MA 02451
Phone: 781-890-0220
Fax: 781-890-2411
Website: www.familyaware.org
E-mail: info@familyaware.org

Helpguide

Website: www.helpguide.org

International Foundation for Research and Education on Depression

P.O. Box 17598
Baltimore, MD 21297
Fax: 443-782-0739
Website: www.ifred.org
E-mail: info@ifred.org

International OCD Foundation

P.O. Box 961029
Boston, MA 02196
Phone: 617-973-5801
Fax: 617-973-5803
Website: www.ocfoundation.org
E-mail: info@ocfoundation.org

International Society for the Study of Trauma and Dissociation (ISSTD)

8400 Westpark Dr.
Second Fl.
McLean, VA 22102
Phone: 703-610-9037
Fax: 703-610-0234
Website: www.isst-d.org
E-mail: info@isst-d.org

International Society for Traumatic Stress Studies

One Parkview Plaza
Ste. 800
Oakbrook Terr., IL 60181
Phone: 847-686-2234
Fax: 847-686-2251
Website: www.istss.org
E-mail: istss@istss.org

Kristin Brooks Hope Center (KBHC)

1250 24th St. N.W., Ste. 300
Washington, DC 20037
Phone: 202-536-3200
Fax: 202-536-3206
Website: www.hopeline.com

Mental Health America (formerly National Mental Health Association)

500 Montgomery St., Ste. 820
Alexandria, VA 22314
Toll-Free: 800-969-6642
Phone: 703-684-7722
Fax: 703-684-5968
Website: www.mentalhealthamerica.net

Mental Health Minute

Website: www.mentalhealthminute.info

Mind

15–19 Bdwy.
Stratford, London, UK E15 4BQ
Phone: +44 208-519-2122
Fax: +44 208-522-1725
Website: www.mind.org.uk
E-mail: supporterservices@mind.org.uk

National Alliance on Mental Illness (NAMI)

3803 N. Fairfax Dr., Ste. 100
Arlington, VA 22203
Toll-Free: 888-999-NAMI (888-999-6264)
/ Toll-Free: 800-950-NAMI (800-950-6264 Helpline)
Phone: 703-524-7600
Fax: 703-524-9094
Website: www.nami.org
E-mail: info@nami.org

National Association of Anorexia Nervosa and Associated Disorders (ANAD)

220 N. Green St.
Chicago, IL 60607
Phone: 630-577-1333
Helpline: 630-577-1330
Website: www.anad.org
E-mail: supportgroups@anad.org

National Association of School Psychologists (NASP)

4340 E. W. Hwy, Ste. 402
Bethesda, MD 20814
Toll-Free: 866-331-NASP (866-331-6277)
Phone: 301-657-0270
TTY: 301-657-4155
Fax: 301-657-0275
Website: www.nasponline.org
E-mail: membership@naspweb.org

National Center for Child Traumatic Stress (NCCTS)

Duke University
1121 W. Chapel Hill St., Ste. 201
Durham, NC 27701
Phone: 919-682-1552
Fax: 919-613-9898
Website: www.nctsn.org
E-mail: info@nctsn.org

National Center for Posttraumatic Stress Disorder (NCPTSD)

U.S. Department of Veterans Affairs (VA)
810 Vermont Ave. N.W.
Washington, DC 20420
Toll-Free: 844-698-2311
Website: www.va.gov

National Center for Victims of Crime (NCVC)

2000 M St. N.W., Ste. 480
Washington, DC 20036
Phone: 202-467-8700
Fax: 202-467-8701
Website: www.ncvc.org
E-mail: webmaster@ncvc.org

National Council on Problem Gambling

730 11th St. N.W., Ste. 601
Washington, DC 20001
Toll-Free: 800-522-4700 (Hotline)
Phone 202-547-9204
Fax: 202-547-9206
Website: www.ncpgambling.org
E-mail: ncpg@ncpgambling.org

National Eating Disorders Association (NEDA)

200 W. 41st St., Ste. 1203
New York, NY 10036
Toll-Free: 800-931-2237
Phone: 212-575-6200
Fax: 212-575-1650
Website: www.nationaleatingdisorders.org
E-mail: info@NationalEatingDisorders.org

National Federation of Families for Children's Mental Health

12320 Parklawn Dr.
Rockville, MD 20852
Phone: 240-403-1901
Fax: 240-403-1909
Website: www.ffcmh.org
E-mail: ffcmh@ffcmh.org

National Institute of Mental Health (NIMH)

6001 Executive Blvd.
Bethesda, MD 20892
Toll-Free: 866-615-6464
Phone: 301-443-4536
Toll-Free TTY: 866-415-8051
TTY: 301-443-8431
Fax: 301-443-4279
Website: www.nimh.nih.gov
E-mail: nimhinfo@nih.gov

National Institute on Alcohol Abuse and Alcoholism (NIAAA)

5635 Fishers Ln.
Rm. 2005, MSC 9304
Bethesda, MD 20892
Phone: 301-443-2857
Website: www.niaaa.nih.gov
E-mail: NIAAAPressOffice@mail.nih.gov

National Institute on Drug Abuse (NIDA)

6001 Executive Blvd.
Rm. 5213, MSC 9561
Bethesda, MD 20892
Phone: 301-443-1124
Fax: 301-443-7397
Website: www.nida.nih.gov and www.drugabuse.gov
E-mail: information@nida.nih.gov

National Women's Health Information Center (NWHIC)

Office on Women's Health (OWH)
200 Independence Ave. S.W.
Rm. 712E
Washington, DC 20201
Toll-Free: 800-994-9662
Phone: 202-690-7650
Toll-Free TDD: 888-220-5446
Fax: 202-205-2631
Website: www.womenshealth.gov

Office of Minority Health (OMH)

Resource Center
P.O. Box 37337
Washington, DC 20013-7337
Toll-Free: 800-444-6472
Phone: 240-453-2882
TDD: 301-251-1432
Fax: 301-251-2160
Website: www.minorityhealth.hhs.gov
E-mail: info@minorityhealth.hhs.gov

Psych Central

55 Pleasant St., Ste. 207
Newburyport, MA 01950
Website: www.psychcentral.com
E-mail: talkback@psychcentral.com

Psychology Today

115 E. 23rd St.
Ninth Fl.
New York, NY 10010
Phone: 212-260-7210
Fax: 212-260-7566
Website: www.psychologytoday.com

Schizophrenic.com

Website: www.schizophrenic.com
E-mail: info@deepdivemedia.net

Social Phobia/Social Anxiety Association
Website: www.socialphobia.org

Substance Abuse and Mental Health Services Administration (SAMHSA)
5600 Fishers Ln.
Rockville, MD 20857
Toll-Free: 877-SAMHSA-7 (877-726-4727)
TTY: 800-487-4889
Fax: 240-221-4292
Website: www.mentalhealth.samhsa.gov

Suicide Awareness Voices of Education (SAVE)
8120 Penn Ave. S.
Ste. 470
Bloomington, MN 55431
Phone: 952-946-7998
Website: www.save.org
E-mail: save@save.org

Suicide Prevention Resource Center (SPRC)
Education Development Center, Inc.
43 Foundry Ave.
Waltham, MA 02453-8313
Toll-Free: 877-GET-SPRC (877-438-7772)
TTY: 617-964-5448
Fax: 617-969-9186
Website: www.sprc.org
E-mail: info@sprc.org

SupportGroups.com
Website: www.supportgroups.com
E-mail: info@supportgroups.com

State Mental Health Resources

Alabama
Division of Mental Health and Substance Abuse Services
Alabama Department of Mental Health
100 N. Union St.
Montgomery, AL 36130-1410
Toll-Free: 800-367-0955 (Hotline)
Phone: 334-242-3454
Fax: 334-242-0725
Website: www.mh.alabama.gov/sa
E-mail: Alabama.DMH@mh.alabama.gov

Arizona
Behavioral Health Services
Arizona Department of Health Services
150 N. 18th Ave.
Ste. 200
Phoenix, AZ 85007
Phone: 602-542-1025
Fax: 602-542-0883
Website: www.azdhs.gov

Arkansas

Division of Behavioral Health Services
Arkansas Department of Human Services
Donaghey Plaza
P.O. Box 1437
Little Rock, AR 72203
Phone: 501-682-1001
TDD: 501-682-8820
Website: www.humanservices.arkansas.gov/
dbhs/Pages/default.aspx

Colorado

Office of Behavioral Health
Department of Human Services
1575 Sherman St.
Eighth Fl.
Denver, CO. 80203-1714
Phone: 303-866-5700
Fax: 303-866-5563
Website: www.colorado.gov/cs/
Satellite/CDHS-BehavioralHealth/
CBON/1251578892077
E-mail: cdhs.communications@state.co.us

Connecticut

Department of Mental Health and
Addiction Services
410 Capitol Ave.
P.O Box 341431
Hartford, CT 06134
Toll-Free: 800-446-7348
Phone: 860-418-7000
TDD: 860-418-6707
Website: www.ct.gov/dmhas
E-mail: DMHAS Webmaster@po.state.ct.us

Delaware

Division of Substance Abuse and Mental
Health
Community Mental Health and Addiction
Services
1901 N. DuPont Hwy
New Castle, DE 19720
Toll-Free: 800-652-2929 (Helpline—
Delaware Only)
Phone: 302-255-9399
Fax: 302-255-4427
Website: www.dhss.delaware.gov/dsamh/
index.html

District of Columbia

Department of Mental Health
64 New York Ave. N.E., Third Fl.
Washington, DC 20002
Phone: 202-673-2200
TTY: 202-673-7500
Fax: 202- 673-3433
Website: www.dmh.dc.gov
E-mail: dbh@dc.gov

Florida

ACCESS Central Mail Center
P.O. Box 1770
Ocala, FL 34478-1770
Toll-Free: 800-962-2873
Toll-Free TTY: 800-453-5145
Website: www.myflfamilies.com/service-
programs/mental-health

Georgia

Division of Addictive Diseases
Department of Behavioral Health and
Developmental Disabilities
Two Peachtree St. N.W.
24th Fl.
Atlanta, GA 30303
Toll-Free: 800-715-4225 (Hotline)
Phone: 404-657-2331
Fax: 404-657-2256
Website: www.dbhdd.georgia.gov

Hawaii

Department of Health
Child and Adolescent Mental Health
Division
3627 Kilauea Ave.
Rm. 101
Honolulu, HI 96816
Phone: 808-733-9333
Fax: 808-733-9357
Website: www.health.hawaii.gov/camhd

Idaho

Division of Behavioral Health
Department of Health and Welfare
P.O. Box 83720
Boise, ID 83720-0036
Toll-Free: 800-922-3406 (Screening/
Referral)
Phone: 208-334-6997
Website: www.healthandwelfare.idaho.gov
E-mail: DPHInquiries@dhw.idaho.gov

Illinois

Division of Alcoholism and Addiction
Department of Human Services
100 S. Grand Ave. E.
Springfield, IL 62762
Toll-Free: 800-843-6154 (Help Line)
Phone: 312-814-5050
Toll-Free TTY: 800-447-6404 (Help Line)
TTY: 312-793-2354
Website: www.dhs.state.il.us/page.
aspx?item=29728
E-mail: DHSWebBits@illinois.gov

Indiana

Division of Mental Health and Addiction
Family and Social Services Administration
402 W. Washington St.
P.O. Box 7083
Indianapolis, IN 46207-7083
Toll-Free: 800-901-1133; 800-662-4357
(Hotline)
Phone: 317-233-4454
Fax: 317-233-4693
Website: www.in.gov/fssa/dmha/index.htm

Iowa

Division of Behavioral Health
Department of Public Health
Lucas State Office Bldg.
321 E. 12th St.
Des Moines, IA 50319-0075
Toll-Free: 866-227-9878
Phone: 515-281-8465
Fax: 515-281-4535
Website: www.idph.state.ia.us/bh/
substance_abuse.asp

Kansas

Community Services and Programs
Department for Aging and Disability
Services
New England State Office Bldg.
555 S. Kansas Ave.
Topeka, KS 66603
Phone: 785-296-3271
Fax: 785-296-5666
Website: www.dcf.ks.gov/Pages/Default.aspx

Kentucky

Cabinet for Health and Family Services
Department for Behavioral Health,
Developmental, and Intellectual Disabilities
275 E. Main St.
4WF
Frankfort, KY 40621
Phone: 502-564-4527
TTY: 502-564-5777
Fax: 502-564-5478
Website: www.dbhdid.ky.gov/kdbhdid/default.aspx

Louisiana

Office of Behavioral Health
Department of Health and Hospitals
P.O. Box 629
Baton Rouge, LA 70821-0629
Phone: 225-342-9500
Fax: 225-342-5568
Website: www.dhh.louisiana.gov/index.cfm/subhome/10/n/6

Maine

Substance Abuse and Mental Health Services
Department of Health and Human Services
41 Anthony Ave.
#11 State House Stn
Augusta, ME 04333-0011
Phone: 207-287-2595
Fax: 207-287-4334
Website: www.maine.gov/dhhs/samhs/osa
E-mail: osa.ircosa@maine.gov

Maryland

Department of Health and Mental Hygiene
201 W. Preston St.
Baltimore, MD 21201
Toll-Free: 877-463-3464
Phone: 410-767-6500
Website: www.dhmh.maryland.gov/bhd/SitePages/Home.aspx
E-mail: dhmh.healthmd@maryland.gov

Massachusetts

Health and Human Services
Office of Children, Youth, and Family
Services
One Ashburton Pl.
11th Fl.
Boston, MA 02108
Phone: 617-573-1600
Website: www.mass.gov/eohhs/consumer/behavioral-health/mental-health

Michigan

Department of Community Health
Capitol View Bldg.
201 Townsend St.
Lansing, MI 48913
Phone: 517-241-2064
Fax: 517-335-8297
Website: www.michigan.gov/mdch
E-mail: hpac@michigan.gov

Minnesota

Department of Human Services
Mental Health Division
P.O. Box 64981
St. Paul, MN 55164-0981
Phone: 651-431-2225
Fax: 651-431-7418
Website: www.mn.gov/dhs
E-mail: Dhs.ChildrensMentalHealth@
state.mn.us

Mississippi

Mississippi Department of Mental Health
1101 Robert E. Lee Bldg.
239 N. Lamar St.
Jackson, MS 39201
Toll-Free: 877-210-8513 (Helpline)
Phone: 601-359-1288
TDD: 601-359-6230
Fax: 601-359-6295
Website: www.dmh.ms.gov

Missouri

Division of Behavioral Health
Missouri Department of Mental Health
P.O. Box 687
Jefferson City, MO 65102
Toll-Free: 800-575-7480
Phone: 573-751-4942
Fax: 573-751-7814
Website: www.dmh.mo.gov/ada
E-mail: dbhmail@dmh.mo.gov

Montana

Addictive and Mental Disorders Division
Department of Public Health and Human
Services
P.O. Box 202905
Helena, MT 59620-2905
Phone: 406-444-3964
Fax: 406-444-9389
Website: www.dphhs.mt.gov/amdd
E-mail: hhsamdemail@mt.gov

Nebraska

Division of Behavioral Health
Department of Health and Human Services
P.O. Box 95026
Lincoln, NE 68509-5026
Toll-Free: 888-866-8660 (Helpline)
Phone: 402-471-8553
Fax: 402-471-9449
Website: www.dhhs.ne.gov/Behavioral_
Health
E-mail: DHHS.HIPAAOffice@nebraska.
gov

Nevada

Department of Health and Human Services
Division of Mental Health and
Development Services
1830 E. College Pkwy.
Ste. 120
Carson City, NV 89706
Phone: 775-684-2940
Fax: 775-684-2949
Website: www.mhds.state.nv.us
E-mail: nmhd@mhd.state.nv.us

New Hampshire

Department of Health and Human Services
105 Pleasant St.
Concord, NH 03301
Toll-Free: 800-804-0909
Phone: 603-271-6738
Fax: 603-271-6105
Website: www.dhhs.nh.gov/index.htm

New Jersey

Department of Human Services
Division of Mental Health and Addiction
Services
222 S. Warren St.
Trenton, NJ 08625
Toll-Free: 800-238-2333 (Hotline)
Phone: 609-292-5760
Fax: 609-292-3816
Website: www.state.nj.us/humanservices/
das/home
E-mail: dmhas@dhs.state.nj.us

New Mexico

Behavioral Health Services Division
Human Services Department
P.O. Box 2348
Santa Fe, NM 87504
Toll-Free: 800-362-2013
Phone: 505-476-9266
Fax: 505-476-9277
Website: www.hsd.state.nm.us/bhsd

New York

State Office of Mental Health
44 Holland Ave.
Albany, NY 12229
Toll-Free: 800-597-8481
Phone: 518-474-6587
Fax: 518-402-4401
Website: www.omh.ny.gov

North Carolina

Department of Health and Human Services
Division of Mental Health, Developmental
Disabilities, and Substance Abuse Services
3007 Mail Service Center
Raleigh, NC 27699-3007
Toll-Free: 800-662-7030
Phone: 919-733-4670
Fax: 919-575-7260
Website: www.dhhs.state.nc.us/mhddsas

North Dakota

Division of Mental Health and Substance
Abuse Services
Department of Human Services
1237 W. Divide Ave.
Ste. 1C
Bismarck, ND 58501-1208
Toll-Free: 800-755-2719 (North Dakota
only)
Phone: 701-328-8920
Fax: 701-328-8969
Website: www.nd.gov/dhs/services/
mentalhealth
E-mail: dhsbhd@nd.gov

Ohio

Department of Mental Health and
Addiction Services
30 E. Broad St.
36th Fl.
Columbus, OH 43215-3430
Toll-Free: 877-275-6364
Phone: 614-466-2596
Toll-Free TTY: 888-636-4889
TTY: 614-752-9696
Fax: 614-752-9453
Website: www.mha.ohio.gov

Oklahoma

Department of Mental Health and
Substance Abuse Services
1200 N.E. 13th St.
P.O. Box 53277
Oklahoma City, OK 73152-3277
Toll-Free: 800-522-9054
Phone: 405-522-3908
TDD: 405-522-3851
Fax: 405-522-3650
Website: www.ok.gov/odmhsas

Oregon

Addictions and Mental Health Division
Oregon Health Authority
500 Summer St. N.E.
Salem, OR 97301-1079
Phone: 503-945-5763
Toll-Free TTY: 800-375-2863
Fax: 503-378-8467
Website: www.oregon.gov/oha/amh/Pages/
index.aspx
E-mail: Amh.web@state.or.us

Pennsylvania

Department of Health
02 Kline Plaza
Ste. B
Harrisburg, PA 17104-1579
Phone: 717-787-4779
Fax: 717-772-0232
Website: www.health.state.pa.us/bdap
E-mail: ra-dhddc@pa.gov

Rhode Island

Department of Behavioral Healthcare
Developmental Disabilities and Hospitals
Barry Hall Bldg.
14 Harrington Rd.
Cranston, RI 02920
Phone: 401-462-2339
Fax: 401-462-3204
Website: www.bhddh.ri.gov/SA

South Carolina

Department of Mental Health
Administration Bldg.
2414 Bull St.
Columbia, SC 29202
Phone: 803- 898-8581
TTY: 864-297-5130
Website: www.state.sc.us/dmh

South Dakota

Division of Community Behavioral Health
Department of Social Services
c/o 700 Governor's Dr.
Pierre, SD 57501
Toll-Free: 800-265-9684
Phone: 605-773-3123
Fax: 605-773-7076
Website: www.dss.sd.gov/
behavioralhealthservices/community

Tennessee

Department of Mental Health and
Substance Abuse Services
601 Mainstream Dr.
Ste. 401
Nashville, TN 37243
Toll-Free: 800-560-5767
Phone: 615-532-6500
Fax: 615-532-6514
Website: www.tn.gov/mental
E-mail: OC.TDMHSAS@tn.gov

Texas

Mental Health and Substance Abuse
Division
Department of State Health Services
P.O. Box 149347
Austin, TX 78714-9347
Toll-Free: 866-378-8440
Phone: 512-206-5000
Fax: 512-206-5714
Website: www.dshs.state.tx.us/MHSA
E-mail: contact@dshs.state.tx.us

Utah

Division of Substance Abuse and Mental
Health
Utah Department of Human Services
195 N. 1950 W.
Salt Lake City, UT 84116
Phone: 801-538-3939
Fax: 801-538-9892
Website: www.dsamh.utah.gov
E-mail: dsamh@utah.gov

Vermont

Department of Mental Health
Redstone Bldg.
26 Terrace St.
Montpelier, VT 05609-1101
Toll-Free: 888-212-4677
Phone: 802-828-3824
Fax: 802-828-3823
Website: www.mentalhealthvermont.gov/
contact

Virginia

Department of Behavioral Health and
Developmental Services
P.O. Box 1797
Richmond, VA 23218-1797
Phone: 804-786-3906
TDD: 804-371-8977
Fax: 804-786-9248
Website: www.dbhds.virginia.gov

Washington

Division of Behavioral Health and Recovery
Services
Department of Social and Health Services
P.O. Box 45330
Olympia, WA 98504-5330
Toll-Free: 877-301-4557
Toll-Free: 866-789-1511 (Help Line)
Toll-Free TTY: 800-833-6384
TTY: 206-461-3219 (Help Line)
Fax: 360-586-0341
Website: www.dshs.wa.gov/dbhr
E-mail: DASAInformation@dshs.wa.gov

West Virginia

Bureau for Behavioral Health and Health
Facilities
Department of Health and Human
Resources
350 Capitol St.
Rm. 350
Charleston, WV 25301
Phone: 304-356-4811
Fax: 304-558-1008
Website: www.dhhr.wv.gov/bhhf/Pages/
default.aspx

Wisconsin

Department of Health Services
One W. Wilson St.
Madison, WI 53703
Toll-Free: 800-947-3529
Phone: 608-266-1865
Website: www.dhs.wisconsin.gov/
MentalHealth/INDEX.HTM

Wyoming

Behavioral Health Division
Mental Health and Substance Abuse
Services
Department of Health, 6101 Yellowstone
Rd.
Ste. 220
Cheyenne, WY 82002
Toll-Free: 800-535-4006
Phone: 307-777-6494
Fax: 307-777-5849
Website: www.health.wyo.gov/
behavioralhealth

Canadian Mental Health Resources

Canadian Mental Health Association

Phoenix Professional Bldg.
595 Montreal Rd. Ste. 303
Ottawa, ON K1K 4L2
Phone: 613-745-7750
Fax: 613-745-5522
Website: www.cmha.ca
E-mail: info@cmha.ca

Canadian Psychological Association

141 Laurier Ave. W. Ste. 702
Ottawa, ON K1P 5J3
Toll-Free: 888-472-0657
Phone: 613-237-2144
Fax: 613-237-1674
Website: www.cpa.ca
E-mail: cpa@cpa.ca

ConnexOntario

685 Richmond St.
London ON N6A 5M1
Phone: 519-439-0174
Fax: 519-439-0455
Toll-Free: 866-531-2600
Website: www.connexontario.ca

Consumers' Health Awareness Network Newfoundland And Labrador (CHANNAL)

284 Lemarchant Rd.
St. John's, NL A1E 1R2
Phone: 753-2560
Toll-Free 1-855- 753-2560
Fax: 709-753-1109
E-mail: admin@channal.ca
Website: www.channal.ca

Healthy Minds Canada

1920 Yonge St., Ste. 300
Toronto, ON M4S 3E2
Phone: 416-351-7757
Toll-Free: 800-915-2773
E-mail: admin@healthymindscanada.ca
Website: www.healthymindscanada.ca

Mental Health First Aid (MHFA) Canada

350 Albert St., Ste. 1210
Ottawa, ON K1R 1A4
Toll-Free: 866-989-3985
Fax: 613-683-3900
E-mail: mhfa@mentalhealthcommission.ca
Website: www.mentalhealthfirstaid.ca

Index

Index

Page numbers that appear in *Italics* refer to tables or illustrations. Page numbers that have a small 'n' after the page number refer to citation information shown as Notes. Page numbers that appear in **Bold** refer to information contained in boxes within the chapters.

N

stepparents, getting along 363
stigma, mental illness 32
"Stigma And Mental Illness" (CDC) 27n
stimulants
    attention deficit hyperactivity disorder 239
    described 291
Strattera (atomoxetine), attention deficit hyperactivity disorder 292
stress
    coping with stress 335
    mental health and wellness 4, 21
    mental illness 330
    psychotherapies 271
    resilience 23
    trauma 342
stress hormones, teen brain 13, **14**
substance abuse
    antisocial personality disorder 114
    delusional disorder 135
    eating disorders 169
    posttraumatic stress disorder 93
Substance Abuse and Mental Health Services Administration (SAMHSA)
    contact 397
    publications
        building self-esteem 321n
        mental health 3n
        warning signs of mental illness 35n
suicide
    bipolar disorder 75
    borderline personality disorder 117
    children and adolescents 39
    depression 29
    prevention 373
Suicide Awareness Voices of Education (SAVE), contact 397
"Suicide In America: Frequently Asked Questions (2015)" (NIMH) 373n
Suicide Lifeguard, mobile app 384
Suicide Prevention Resource Center (SPRC), contact 397
Suicide Safety Plan, mobile app 384
support groups
    anorexia 170
    attention deficit hyperactivity disorder 241
    bipolar disorder 80
    schizophrenia 148
    social anxiety disorder 88
SupportGroups.com, contact 397

synapses, brain 12
Systems Training for Emotional Predictability and Problem Solving (STEPPS), borderline personality disorder 121

T

talk therapy *see* psychotherapy
tardive dyskinesia, antipsychotics 295
"The Teen Brain: 6 Things To Know" (NIMH) 11n
"The Teen Brain: Still Under Construction" (NIMH) 11n
"Teen Dating Violence" (CDC) 221n
Tegretol (carbamazepine), anticonvulsant 296
Tennessee, mental health resource 403
Texas, mental health resource 404
therapists
    anorexia 170
    attention deficit hyperactivity disorder 240
    binge eating disorder 177
    borderline personality disorder 121
    bulimia 174
    Tourette syndrome 246
    see also psychotherapy
Thorazine (chlorpromazine), typical antipsychotics 293
thought disorders, schizophrenia 148
Thursday's Child National Youth Advocacy Hotline, help and hotlines 386
tics, Tourette syndrome 243
TMS (transcranial magnetic stimulation), described 307
Tourette syndrome
    attention deficit hyperactivity disorder 246
    described 243
Tragedy Assistance Program for Survivors (TAPS), help and hotlines 387
traumatic events
    overview 341–5
    resilience 23
"Treating Disruptive Behavior Disorders In Children And Teens" (AHRQ) 197n
treatment
    anorexia 170
    antisocial personality disorder 114
    attention deficit hyperactivity disorder 238
    autism spectrum disorder 233
    binge eating disorder 177
    bipolar disorder 78